Praise for *I Love a Cop*

"A moving, thorough, and honest resource for anyone who knows and/ or loves a law enforcement officer. Whether you 'belong' to a rookie or veteran officer, Dr. Kirschman's matter-of-fact style of laying out situations, facts, and solutions is sure to provide you with a valuable source of information."
> —*Partners Off Duty* newsletter

"An excellent gift to any individual with a family member or loved one who is working in law enforcement. Highly recommended."
> —Fred R. Egloff, Law Enforcement Memorial Association

"When I was Police Chief in Toronto, every graduating police officer received a copy of *I Love a Cop*. This is a 'must read' for all progressive police leaders who really care about officers and their families."
> —David Boothby, chief of police (retired),
> Toronto, Ontario, Canada

"There is finally a training manual on how to survive in a law enforcement family. Reading this book could very well save a few police marriages."
> —Karen Lippe, President, Grand Lodge Auxiliary,
> Fraternal Order of Police

"Police administrators should seriously consider making it required reading for promotional examinations."
> —*FBI Magazine*

"Living with a cop and not understanding what he or she goes through is like riding rapids down the Arkansas River without a raft. This book is long overdue!"
—Suzie Sawyer, Executive Director, Concerns of Police Survivors

"'Must' reading for police recruits, police officers, and their family members."
—Gary Kaufmann, PsyD, Chief Police Psychologist, Michigan Department of State Police

"*I Love a Cop* is a gift of inestimable value to the families themselves, and to the mental health professionals who are attempting to understand and help them."
—Emily B. Visher, PhD, and John S. Visher, MD, Cofounders, Stepfamily Association of America

"Dr. Kirschman's book will be an invaluable tool for the Metro-Dade Police Department, both for training purposes with recruits and for in-service officers."
—Scott W. Allen, PhD, Staff Psychologist, Metro-Dade Police Department, Florida

"A practical coping guide for police officers and the people who love them. Most highly recommended."
—*NJ Cops: New Jersey's Law Enforcement Journal*

"This book breaks through the stereotypes and reaches a 'human' level. . . ."
—*The California Peace Officers Association Network Newsletter*

"This is a great book! My husband is a rookie cop and I found the book extremely helpful. I'm recommending it to all the other cop spouses and family members I know!"
—Liesa M. Persaud, Tulsa, Oklahoma

I LOVE A COP

I LOVE A COP

What Police Families Need to Know
Revised Edition

Ellen Kirschman, PhD

THE GUILFORD PRESS
New York   London

© 2007 Ellen Kirschman
Published by The Guilford Press
A Division of Guilford Publications, Inc.
72 Spring Street, New York, NY 10012
www.guilford.com

Printed in the United States of America

This book is printed on acid-free paper.

Last digit is print number: 9 8 7 6 5 4 3 2 1

Library of Congress Cataloging-in-Publication Data

Kirschman, Ellen.
  I love a cop : what police families need to know / by Ellen
Kirschman. — Rev. ed.
      p. cm.
  Includes bibliographical references and index.
  ISBN-10: 1-59385-353-X   ISBN-13: 978-1-59385-353-2 (pbk.)
  ISBN-10: 1-59385-354-8   ISBN-13: 978-1-59385-354-9 (hardcover)
 1. Police—Job stress. 2. Police—Family relationships.
3. Police psychology. I. Title.
  HV7936.J63K57 2006
  363.201'9—dc22
                                                      2006012306

This book is dedicated
to the men and women of law enforcement
and their families

ACKNOWLEDGMENTS

The following list of acknowledgments is much shorter than it would be if I could openly thank all the cops and police families who generously shared their private experiences because they believed that doing so would help other cops and their families. Privacy is a hallmark of the police culture; most cops do not readily share secrets with outsiders. The men and women who have permitted me to use their stories have demonstrated courage and generosity beyond the call of duty.

I couldn't have fully addressed the wide range of topics affecting police families without the bountiful counsel and encouragement of hardworking friends and professional colleagues who found the time to return phone calls, send papers, cite reference material, introduce me to people I could interview, and read drafts of the book: Jim Anderson, PhD; Carole Ballachey, PhD; Joanne Bellow, LCSW; Greg Bellow, PhD; Jules Bernstein, Esq.; Lt. Al Benner, PhD, Sgt. Forrest Fulton, PhD, and Sgt. Vicki Quinn, San Francisco Police Department; Sgt. Mike Boggess and Lt. Walt Tibbet, San Jose Police Department; Nancy Bohl, PhD; Leanor Boulin-Johnson, PhD, Arizona State University; Robin Buhrke, PhD, Duke University; Janet Childs, The Center for Living with Dying; Katherine Czesak, PhD; Claire D'Agostino, PhD, and Gregory Swann, PhD, Atlanta Police Department; Bill Feister, PhD; Richard Gelles, PhD; Kevin Gilmartin, PhD; Susan Hanks, PhD, California School of Professional Psychology; Ret. Chief

Acknowledgments

Penny Harrington, National Center for Women and Policing; Celia Heady, Idaho Council on Domestic Violence; Lt. Chris Hetherington, Officer Lydia Martinez, and St. Kevin Walsh, New York Police Department; Audrey Honig, PhD, Los Angeles Sheriffs Department; Paula Lundberg-Love, PhD, University of Texas; Coleen McGrath, New York State Office for the Prevention of Domestic Violence; Peter Neidig, PhD; Ann O'Dell, San Diego Police Department (retired); Gary Olson, PhD; Jim Reese, PhD, FBI (retired) and the Behavioral Science Unit of the FBI; Hal Russell, PhD; Susan Saxe-Clifford, PhD; Suzie Sawyer, COPS; Guy Schiller, MA; Ellen Scrivner, PhD; Chuck Stewart, PhD; Sandra Stith, PhD, Virginia Polytechnic Institute; Phil Trompetter, PhD; John Violanti, PhD, Rochester Institute of Technology; Emily Visher, PhD; John Visher, MD; and Officer Mark Wynn, Nashville Police Department. I am also indebted to the work of Harriet Goldhor Lerner, PhD, whose self-help books served as models for my own.

I am indebted as well to colleagues who helped with this revised edition: Suzanne Best, PhD, Steve Curran, PhD, Robyn Gershon, PhD, Mike Roberts, PhD, John Violanti, PhD, and Craig Weisman, PhD, my colleagues on the IACP listserv, and Lorraine Greene, PhD, who was my partner in developing policefamilies.com.

There are several people whose faith and trust in me formed the foundation from which this book was ultimately launched: Ruth Nagler, Georgi La Berge, and Canada College sponsored the first "I Love a Cop" class in 1977; my teachers, Verneice Thompson, PhD, and Charles Hampden-Turner, PhD, taught me to see beyond the obvious; and the men and women of the Palo Alto Police Department hired me as a consultant right out of graduate school in 1983 and have been putting up with me ever since.

I am fortunate to have worked with the staff at The Guilford Press. This book was a leap for them, and they put their hearts into it. My editor, Kitty Moore, treated me and the book with careful consideration and extended her friendship, as well as her expertise. Sarah Lavender Smith gave the revision a careful reading. Her suggestions have made this a better book.

Finally, I have what we all need: a supportive, loving family. My father, Lewis, loved books but sadly didn't live to see this one. My mother, Dorothy, who died in 1999, was my greatest fan, and my brother, Richard, continues to be an endless source of laughter and ideas; Steve Johnson, who is now my husband, gave me much to look forward to and made the isolation of writing easier to bear; and my sister-in-law/friend/writing coach, Doris Ober, is a principled, tough, and talented editor whose guidance has been indispensable from beginning to end.

CONTENTS

INTRODUCTION

It would be hard to imagine a job more written
about, and less understood, than that of a cop. The
cop's world has been combed over by novelists,
playwrights, screenwriters, television producers, and
the inquisitive press, yet the practitioner and close
observer knows that the world occupied by America's
cops remains *terra incognita*.
—RET. CHIEF ANTHONY BOUZA

I was attending an orientation session for families of new officers
and dispatchers. The room was crowded with people: spouses,
children, mothers, fathers, stepparents, siblings, fiancées, and significant others. The children were dressed in Sunday-school best.
Everyone looked nervous and happy at the same time. They were,
I think, a little puzzled at being invited to the police department.
Some of the laterals (cops hired from other agencies) had never
before brought their families to work. The brand new rookies
were too green to realize how unusual this event was.

The agenda for the evening covered a range of topics. The police chief gave a brief welcome. The lieutenant in charge of personnel described the benefits program available to officers and
their families. The officer coordinating field training talked about
the demands of training on the new officers and their families and
the specifics of what was taught. A member of the peer-staffed
critical incident intervention team talked about trauma and what
the department does to provide emotional support to officers involved in critical incidents. Two veteran wives, one a young

mother and the other a grandmother, shared their experiences with the group.

I was last up. It was my job to talk about the myths and realities of police work and the emotional hazards associated with the job. The families listened intently to me, but they were very quiet. I jokingly suggested they had been prompted by their cops not to ask embarrassing questions. I encouraged them to speak out. Their first questions centered on safety issues that were paramount in their minds. But beneath those questions, I sensed other concerns too troubling or embarrassing to raise in public. I tried to talk about those concerns without waiting to be asked. How will this job change the person I love? How will I fare in the struggle for possession of his or her time and attention? How will the excitement of police work compare to the day-to-day tasks of running a family? What happens if my cop grows bitter, cynical, or racist, and we no longer share the same views of the world? What are the chances we'll get divorced?

How could I explain, in the short time allotted to me, that how a police officer and his or her family fares through a 20-year career depends on many things?

- The job itself—meaning the physical, intellectual, and emotional demands of the work
- The amount of control an officer can exert over these demands
- The organizational culture and the leadership style of his or her agency
- The absence or presence of opportunities for career development
- The relationship between the police department and the community
- Individual factors such as the officer's personality and style of coping with stress, the quality and availability of family relationships and support systems, health concerns, and financial stability
- And last, but never least, *luck*

That evening, as I talked about the emotional hazards of police work, I worried that I was raining on everyone's parade. This was an evening to feel proud, happy, and hopeful. It was hard to talk about negative things in the midst of such optimism. What kept me going was my belief that presenting a realistic view of the future is one of the best antidotes to burnout and disappointment. And if it was hard to hear negative talk on a night like this, at least I had mapped out the territory, as I understood it, so that families traveling along this route together would not feel quite so lost when the road got bumpy, as I knew it must.

SPILLOVER

Family orientations are a really good way to acknowledge how important police families are and how much the job will spill over into their private lives. In this era of easy slogans about the sanctity of family life and family values, the truth is that there is little in our society and in our workplaces that supports families. Many of the young children in the room were there because their parents couldn't find adequate, affordable childcare. Most of the spouses worked full time because their families needed two incomes just to keep up. They all had more than they could reasonably do to juggle all their responsibilities as parents, children, spouses, siblings, citizens, friends, and employees.

Tonight was a happy event, but what happens when trouble spills over at home or at work? Instead of being a buffer against stress, family members can become targets for the stress produced at work, or work can become a target for the stress produced at home. There is no realistic way to keep work and family separate; in fact, it may be damaging to try. So what I hoped to do on that night, and in this book, was, and is, to encourage families to act as a team and energetically manage the spillover between work and home.

DIVORCE: MYTHS AND REALITIES

Our society is preoccupied with police work. There are so many television series, docudramas, news broadcasts, and movies about police work that it is nearly impossible to separate the myths

3

from the realities of the job. This was as true for the police officers and families who were in the room that night as it is for the public.

One of the unspoken myths I wanted to discredit is that police marriages are destined for failure because of the job. Marriage and family life are never easy to sustain, regardless of what you or your mate do for a living. There are times, I am sure, when we are all amazed at how families function—how two or more separate human beings with different backgrounds, values, biological and sexual needs, communication styles, and so forth can form an enduring partnership. Even those of us who are partners with someone quite like ourselves know that there are still essential differences between us. And those of us who are attracted to our opposites may come to regret the very thing that drew us to that person in the first place.

What we bring into our adult relationships from our families of origin and our cultural conditioning in terms of expectations, attitudes, self-esteem, needs, and interpersonal skills is as important an influence on family life as is the work we do. Police families and police psychologists often forget this fact and blame too much on the job. It *is* true that habits learned at work, particularly police work, can be hazardous to home life. And certain "givens" of the job, such as the long hours, are not family friendly. But, perhaps the most damaging factor is that police work provides a ready-made scapegoat for a troubled marriage and an easy out for avoiding the task of managing differences with loved ones and learning positive ways to build, strengthen, and maintain a family.

Some years ago, I observed a respected colleague address a large group of police officers, their spouses, and their significant others. He stood on the stage and instructed the cops in the audience to look at the cop to their left, to their right, in front, and in back of them. He then told them that in five years one of them would be divorced and three of them would be unfaithful. At the break, I went to the women's room, where I found any number of women in a state of high anxiety over this preposterous and unverifiable claim. I didn't want to think about the painful conversations that would take place in the car on the way home—all in response to an unsubstantiated myth.

Statistics about divorce in police work are very hard to pin down and are inherently unreliable. Even if these statistics could be verified, they are only meaningful when compared to other occupations, other locales, other cultures. Several police-specific studies suggest that the first three years of marriage are the most precarious and that if a male officer stays married beyond those three years, his marriage is, in fact, more stable than one in the general population. Another way of saying this is that 75% of police officers who get divorced will do so within their first three years on the job. (The rate of divorce among female officers is apparently higher and is discussed in Chapter 12.)

Some researchers go so far as to claim that second marriages of police officers are as strong if not stronger than those in comparison groups. Other studies indicate that the crucial factors in couples at risk for divorce are how young they were when they married and if they married before or after one of them joined the police force.

There are so many variables to be considered in studying divorce that it is simply unwise to infer a cause-and-effect relationship between police work and divorce on the basis of statistics alone.

What about infidelity? The prevalent myth is that cops—male cops particularly—are frequently unfaithful because they have so many opportunities to meet women, and there are so many women who are attracted to cops. Getting dependable facts about people's sexual behavior is difficult to do, and locker-room talk is hardly a reliable source of information. Police work can be used to excuse infidelity, but I think it is closer to the truth to say that infidelity, however often it occurs, is not so much a consequence of the job as it is a reflection of the people involved. (See Chapter 11 for more information on divorce and infidelity.)

HOW TO USE THIS BOOK

When the evening was over and all the pizza eaten, the families filed out the door, shaking hands and saying thanks. Now they had faces to put with names; they had met their mate's training officer in person, talked directly with the critical incident intervention team, and met a psychologist they might one day see again. I thought the evening was successful. I always like getting out of my office because it gives me a chance to get to know more about the officers and families I treat. I get to see the places they work and the communities they serve. I learn something about the quality of their work life and their home life as well.

Readers obviously do not have the same opportunity. Because of that, the kind of advice you will find in this book is general. You will no doubt need to tailor my suggestions to your specific situation. Sometimes you might want to consider getting professional guidance.

The fact that you are reading this book may mean that you are the person in your family who feels responsible for changing things that aren't going well. On the other hand, you may be the person in your family who is most unhappy and most needs things to change. Reading this book will help you think about how to separate what you can change from what you can't.

The stories in this book are drawn from my files and the files of my colleagues in police psychology. All of the characters have been disguised to protect the identity of the individuals involved, except when I have been given permission to use real names. A few are composites—two or more actual stories combined together to preserve anonymity or for clarification. They are drawn from all parts of the country, though many are from the West Coast. Most, though not all, of the subjects work in small- to moderate-sized departments of 50 to 300 cops.

You can use this book in two ways. You can sit down and read it straight through. Not every chapter will apply to your family, of course, but most will apply to someone you know. Or, you can use this book like a medical manual—turning to specific chapters as you need them. You might want to read it together with your loved one—consider it preventive medicine—and make it a springboard for future planning. Families who prepare for the future seem to fare better than those who don't. When you are prepared for what might happen, you feel less isolated and helpless if it does. This is especially so for people who are associated with a career that has so much unpredictable change.

Whether you are new to policing or a veteran spouse, you may find the chapters devoted to trauma to be the toughest part of this book. You can read these chapters if or when you need them, but when something traumatic happens, most people are too "antsy" to sit still and read. If you don't want to read them now, my advice is to skim that section so you know what's there if you need it. I hope you never do.

A NOTE ABOUT THIS REVISED EDITION

I Love a Cop: What Police Families Need to Know was meant to be about the everyday challenges facing police officers and their families throughout their careers. But in the years since it was first published in 1997, there has occurred an extraordinary series of catastrophes, natural and man-made. Although we do not yet know the long-term effects of these disasters, we do know that the law enforcement community has repeatedly shown remarkable courage and resilience in the face of overwhelming danger and tragedy. Unfortunately, there is more to come. The world seems to have grown increasingly dangerous; the ever-present threat of terrorism hovers over all our lives, most especially those of first responders and their families.

I revised *I Love a Cop* in light of this new "normal" without altering the essential material from the first edition. You'll find many changes in the chapters on trauma and resilience, which I expanded to include important new information and tips on disaster preparedness. I enhanced the chapters on domestic abuse and alcohol abuse to reflect recent developments, and I updated most statistics throughout. There are new books on the recommended reading list and new resources in the resource section, including some in the United Kingdom, Canada, and Australia.

Finally, I rededicate this book to law enforcement professionals and their families everywhere for their courage and persistence in the ordinary and extraordinary days to come. Thank you for taking risks so that the rest of us may feel secure.

PART I

"HI, HONEY.
I'M HOME."

CHAPTER 1

THE WAY IT IS

Givens and Realities of Police Work

> How can you be commanding, ordering, and
> directing by day—hiding your emotions, hiding that
> you are afraid . . . and then open the door and say,
> "Hi, Honey. I'm home"?
> —BEVERLY J. ANDERSON, PhD,
> *Director, Metropolitan Police*
> *Employee Assistance Program*

There are certain "givens" in police work: dimensions of the job that probably won't change much. The first is shift work. The second is the long hours. The third is that the work itself is crisis-driven and therefore unpredictable. The fourth is that officers and their families live in the limelight of public scrutiny. The fifth is the physical nature of patrol work and frequency of on-the-job injuries. I have added a sixth since *I Love a Cop* was first published in 1997: separations and long deployments necessitated by disasters, both natural and man-made.

The reactions of Danny's family show how tough it is when the givens mount up. Danny came home in the middle of his shift in the middle of the night, having been badly beaten by a gang of thugs. He was feeling humiliated for losing a "cop toss," as he called it. While he had no broken bones or serious injuries, he was cut, bruised, and frightened. He had nearly lost his weapon in the melee, which had lasted for the longest five minutes of his life. To add insult to injury, after he and his backup officer arrested the gang, they had laughed in his face and promised to sue him for brutality. Because Danny came home unexpectedly, he inadvertently awoke his family. His wife's first reaction was to yell at him for waking their baby, who was colicky and had only just fallen asleep. Danny worked midnights and had put in a lot of overtime that month. Terri was exhausted and irritable most of the time. She was tired of being cooped up at home with no relief and frustrated by trying to keep the baby quiet during the day. In the dark and in her sleepy state, she didn't notice his bruises or bandages. He needed comfort, and what he got was further humiliation.

Danny had to go to court and face his assailants and their families—large, unruly groups of people who followed him down the hall into the bathroom, making obscene gestures and whispered threats. It was all he could do to look at them and testify.

All of this made the news, and Terri couldn't go anywhere without someone asking her what happened. Danny and even Terri's own family hardly wanted to talk about anything else. No one seemed to care how she was managing with a colicky child and an injured husband.

Because no shots had been fired or bones broken, Danny's department virtually ignored his experience and his injuries. Typically for a cop, he felt too ashamed of losing the fight to ask for help. His physical injuries healed quickly, but his emotional injuries persisted until he developed ulcers and a highly reactive patrol style that finally got some attention from his superiors, who gave him a modified duty assignment and referred him for counseling.

SHIFT WORK

Shift workers in general are set apart from mainstream American life. We all grow up with expectations based on our own families of origin and on cultural images of the ordinary family delivered by the media. It is sometimes a shock to realize how far from ordinary the life of a cop's family can be.

Shift work, especially the midnight shift, is difficult and disrupts normal sleep patterns. It's hard to stay up with the family on days off. Graveyard officers are vulnerable to overusing alcohol and sedatives to get to sleep and caffeine and over-the-counter stimulants to stay awake. In some communities the graveyard shift is exciting because many arrests are made at this time, but in low-crime communities staying awake between 2:00 and 6:00 A.M. can be an agonizing effort.

Working "dogwatch" is isolating. One cop told me that as he and his squad drove out of the police garage at night, he felt as though they were all little boats leaving the mother ship, heading out into a vast, dark, and empty ocean.

Swing watch can also be hard on family life. Earl worked swings, and his family was asleep when he got home at 1:00 A.M. He felt lonely coming into a dark, quiet house and needed something to do besides drink and watch old movies on television. He and his wife worked out a routine. When he arrives home now, all the lights are on, so the house looks welcoming. His wife leaves him a news-filled note on the computer. He looks in on his children, puts out the garbage, throws in a load of wash if needed, walks the dog, and makes his kids' school lunches. By the time he's finished, he's ready for sleep. Shifting gears and contributing to domestic tasks help him to feel more like a member of the family than a boarder who pays the bills.

Sleep deprivation takes its toll on work performance, even of the safety-conscious officer. It takes an additional toll on the family members who have the Herculean task of keeping the kids quiet so that mom or dad can sleep during the day. Couples without children find themselves spending more time with friends than they do with each other, and they may sleep alone more than they did when they were single. Single parents may have to resort to recruiting friends and family to help out. The biggest burden falls on those families who are trying to live with a brutal schedule of rotating shifts.

Of course, people differ in their sleep needs. Some people, like Annie, are "night owls" and love being on graveyard. Annie is an independent sort who wants to live in the country, where she can ski and fish. Working dogwatch means she misses the traffic and the "brass." She earns more money with night differential and has arranged her upside-down life to take advantage of the time she spends at home during the day. Night owls are lucky and probably always get their first choice of shift.

Shift work makes planning for weekends, holidays, and social and school events difficult. Non-shift-working friends and family may find it hard to deal with the cop's lack of availability, and friendships may begin to drift apart.

Shift work was the hardest adjustment Sara and Randy had to make when they were married—it required them to be more flexible, creative, and mindful of planning than they had been before. Over the years, they have discovered many hidden benefits. They know shift work has allowed Randy to spend a lot more time with his kids than do many of his friends who work from 9:00 to 5:00.

Randy now works midnights. He has been able to help out at his son's late afternoon soccer practice. He drives his kids to school in the morning. He goes to after-school parent-teacher meetings, even if he misses the school play. When one of the kids is sick, he can stay home with one kid while Sara takes the other one to the doctor. Or, he can stay home with the sick kid, so Sara doesn't have to miss work. He can go to the bank or food shopping, so Sara doesn't have to go on her lunch hour. Occasionally, they get to do things as a couple while the kids are in school.

Over the years, Randy and Sara have learned creative ways to observe holidays. While they both still long to celebrate New Year's Eve together, they settle for a special breakfast instead. They've found their children to be creative planners who love to make up new "traditions" that are unique to their family. The children enjoy exploring their family heritage for ideas about holiday rituals.

Sara and Randy also make good use of available communications technology. They both have Blackberries. (Blackberries are wireless handheld devices with phones.) At home they use Post-It notes to stay in touch. Public safety therapist Guy Shiller thinks cops *love* Post-It notes because they are used to communicating with each other over the air in a short, terse style. One woman told him that when she was feeling frustrated because shift work was interfering with her sex life, she would leave her mate a cryptic Post-It note that said, "Think sex"—a kind of intellectual foreplay!

Because shift work and other givens are part of the job, it is crucial to face them directly as soon as possible and to problem-solve,

---

Tips for Dealing with Shift Work

- If you are scared to be home alone at night, say so. You have every right to feel comfortable and safe in your own home. Consider installing a security alarm, motion detector lights, and locks on the windows and doors. Buy a dog. Make your home and your bedroom an appealing place, where you feel secure when you are by yourself.
- Find other police spouses or families who will be alone at nights or on holidays. Get together with them. If you are a single parent, try finding others and share childcare. Remember there are 12 to 16 nonworking hours left in a day. The whole day is not ruined when your officer has to work.
- Use your alone time to advantage. Think about what stimulates and gratifies you intellectually, emotionally, spiritually, or physically.
- Remind yourself that shift work is temporary; most police departments eventually allow officers to change shifts or to rotate into a fixed-hour specialty. Try to think of a way shift work might be an advantage in the future.
- Make dates with each other. Knowing you and your spouse will have some time alone every Tuesday morning may be the anchor that gets you through the rest of the week.

---

negotiate, and strategize around them. Veteran spouses all warn that fighting, nagging, crying, pleading, and blaming only make you and your cop feel depressed or guilty about something over which neither of you has much control. It is futile to try to change the unchangeable, and it will only alienate the person you most want to be close to. This does not mean you have to suffer in silence.

LONG HOURS

We Americans are an industrious people. The hours we commit to work exceed the hours we spend at home. We are driven by financial need—our dollar does not buy what it did for our parents, and most of us require two incomes to achieve the standard of living our parents earned with one.

We are also ambitious. Our culture rewards us for achievement and accumulation. Men especially are made to feel less than successful if they fail to climb the ladder of achievement, whereas woman are still regarded with skepticism if they appear more devoted to career than family. On the other hand, our workplaces, in general, are not family-friendly; they are designed to reward the employee who is free to devote countless hours to work.

Police work is a "greedy" profession, though certainly not the only one. It demands and rewards long hours. It is the rare police officer who works a 40-hour shift. Special assignments, training, preparing for promotion, court appearances, and overtime all extend the work week. An officer's willingness to work extra hours is subtly reinforced by the organization. Failure to volunteer for overtime assignments may be perceived as not pulling a fair share of the load. Going home rather than hanging out with the "guys" may make a cop seem distant, unfriendly, and perhaps unreliable to his or her coworkers. This puts pressure on officers who believe they won't get backed up on the street if they aren't well liked and "one of the gang."

The officer who asks for time off for family reasons may be unfairly seen as having domestic problems or difficulty keeping his or her home life at home. This is what happened to Sam when his wife, Becky, discovered a lump in her breast. Both she and Sam were terrified. It took days to get to see a doctor and then days more to get the results. Becky was extremely anxious—her aunt had died of breast cancer, and her mother had recently had a mastectomy. She needed Sam with her. Sam was torn. He was still in training and thought it made him look bad to miss work. He didn't want anyone to know what was going on because he didn't want anyone to feel sorry for him. He was so scared that he thought he would cry if anyone asked what was wrong. He never even shared the good news when the lump turned out to be benign.

For cops, dedication to the job, not the family, seems to be the important consideration, both for belonging and for promotion. This is a trap for cops who are convinced that advancement is the only way to better provide for their families and make them proud. It is also a paradox that officers who work long hours in order to get promoted may be so exhausted and limited in the amount of quality time spent at home that they are alienating the very people for whom they are working such long hours. Their families may not appreciate the pay or promotional opportunities associated with special assignments or think these benefits offset the long hours away from home or the increased risk associated with some specialties, such as undercover narcotics work.

It is not just the long hours away that can get to you. Police families everywhere complain that even when their cop is home, he or she is thinking about the job or is preoccupied with organizational politics or ongoing cases. This absorption in the job,

---

Tips for Dealing with the Long Hours

- Make clear verbal agreements about the importance of your family unit and hold each other to these agreements.
- Get everyone to write down a list of priorities. Compare your lists.
- Insist that your mate deal with you and not use the job as an excuse.
- Learn problem-solving techniques (see Recommended Reading in the Resources section) so you can fix the problem, not the blame.
- Talk about what you value in life. If the job is providing you or your spouse with excitement you are missing at home, talk about how you can build more excitement into your personal life.
- Approach differences by fighting both for yourself *and* your relationship. Be a tough bargainer. Relationships do not profit over the long run when one partner is either consistently self-sacrificing or self-interested. If you fail to ensure that your own needs are met, you will have nothing to give anyone else.
- Accept that you may each have different needs for time alone. This may be hard to accept when you have so little time together. Every couple needs to balance their needs for closeness and autonomy.

(cont.)

(continued from previous page)

- Remember that children need quality *and* quantity time with a parent. It is hard to have quality time with children you see infrequently because they need time to warm up to you. Avoid disappointing your children or promising what can't be delivered.
- Take vacations with and without your kids. Try to get away for several long weekends, as well as for a longer trip. Take one "secret vacation" with your spouse and don't tell *anyone* where you're going.
- Set up a regularly scheduled "couple hour" in which you each talk about important issues in your life but neither of you discusses work.
- Do whatever you can to create more time for each other.
- Manage your finances wisely. Sometimes officers work a lot of overtime or take a second job because they and their families have material needs beyond their means. Cops frequently own expensive toys—four-wheel-drive vehicles, speedboats, motorcycles, dirt bikes, big houses in the suburbs, and more. Young officers especially may be overwhelmed by the amount of money they are earning and go on a spending spree, creating instant debt with their instant wealth.
- Consider setting aside a percentage of your collective take-home pay and putting half of that in individual bank accounts so you each have some discretionary money for personal expenses.
- If you blame the job for your unhappiness, you may put your mate on the defensive instead of recruiting him or her as a problem-solving ally. He or she may already be using work as a way to avoid dealing with the friction that exists between you.
- Learn to disagree and fight fairly (see "Recommended Reading"). Learn to tolerate your own anxiety about disagreeing—don't assume it means the end of the relationship.
- Communicate with your mate. If you find yourself telling your friends and relatives about a problem you are having with your mate before you tell your mate, you're probably not communicating well. It's comforting and enlightening to talk with friends and family, but it won't solve the problem you're having at home.

which is usually most intense at the rookie phase, can be a real turn-off to family and friends. It seems as though your cop can't talk about anything else but police work. He or she monopolizes conversations, watches every cop show on television, and provides a running critique on the action to anyone who'll listen. Your interests, your problems, your accomplishments, or those of your friends and family, may pale in comparison.

UNPREDICTABILITY

I once heard someone describe police work as three hours of boredom, followed by two minutes of terror, concluding with six hours of report writing. Every shift is unpredictable because police work is driven by crises and emergency responses. This is alluring, even addicting, to many cops, who love the variety and spontaneity. It's a lot like gambling.

Unpredictability is hard on families because it leads to last-minute changes. Unplanned overtime, being called in for court on a day off (and then having the hearing canceled or postponed), arrests made late in the shift, cases requiring extraordinary paperwork, filling in for a sick officer, and so on all play havoc with a planned schedule and send a message to the family that the job takes priority over their needs.

Jack and Judy learned to problem-solve the management of frequent last-minute changes. They bought a second car and routinely made backup plans in case Judy got stuck at work. They worked out a system of "rain checks" and treated themselves to something special when their plans were canceled at the last minute. Just planning the rain checks took the edge off their mutual disappointment.

Handling these last-minute changes takes time and frank discussion. You may want your cop to telephone you as soon as possible if he or she will be late coming home so you can go on with your plans or change them. You have every right to expect this kind of common courtesy—which is not the same as "reporting" in. If your mate "forgets" to call, you need to let him or her know, in a calm way, that you are hurt and angry and that ignoring your needs is unacceptable and disrespectful of your time.

Scheduling is not the only unpredictable given you will face. It is also hard to predict what kind of mood your loved one will be in at the end of a shift. Will your spouse be coming home exhilarated after a good arrest or depressed because of a poor performance evaluation? Will he or she be bone tired after "shagging" calls without a break or irritable with boredom? While there is a little of the unexpected in many jobs, there is a lot in most emergency response professions.

Police officers are like doctors. The work they do is important, and every action they take may have unpredictable, serious consequences and risks. Officers are keenly aware that what they do can become the object of an internal investigation. Whether that investigation results from a serious infraction or a frivolous complaint, it takes a terrible toll on the officer and his or her family. It is so upsetting to be the object of one of these investigations that the first thought many officers have after a shooting is not "I'm glad to be alive" but "Will this cost me my job?" This apprehension rose appreciably following the Rodney King incident and is still strong today.

Tips for Dealing with Unpredictability

- Stick to your plans even if you have to go on without your mate. We live in a coupled-up world, and it can be awkward to go places alone or unescorted. Develop the ability to go places alone rather than miss out on things that are important to you.
- Pair up with others who may also be alone.
- Try to work out some "homecoming" habits. Homecoming is often the "arsenic hour"—everyone has needs and no one has anything left to give. Everyone unwinds differently: Some like to talk, and some like to retreat. Many cops want to "decompress" on their first day off. They need a break from problems before tackling family concerns and will be happy to talk—but only after they have had a problem-free day to themselves. Learn about each other's needs. Respect your differences.

Your family's financial stability may be heavily, if not totally, dependent on the actions of your police mate, actions over which you have no control. It may be small consolation to remember that contractors, politicians, physicians, and almost all self-employed people run the same risks in that injuries, lawsuits, and catastrophes beyond their control are part of the price of doing business. There are no guarantees anywhere.

PUBLIC SCRUTINY

Police families live in the same limelight cops do. This puts pressure on police families who regard themselves as ordinary as anyone else. If it were not such an invasion of privacy, it would be almost comical to think how police officers are treated like public property. A real estate agent, showing me a house for sale, pointed out that one of the advantages of buying this house was that a police officer lived next door, almost as though he or she was a private security guard for the neighborhood. I wasn't surprised because I have heard countless stories of neighbors banging on an officer's front door during dinner time rather than calling 911.

As a family member or friend, you may feel like an unpaid representative of the police department. After all, it is you who most often attends nonpolice events and gets to bear the brunt of listening to negative opinions about cops or to parry questions about the latest police scandal. At times you may feel defensive and want to withdraw into a circle of police-only folks, or you might find yourself wishing your spouse did something else for a living.

Your children will also take the heat for being part of a police family. They may be held to a higher standard and told that, as police officers' children, they should be better behaved than other kids. Try not to make this same mistake yourself. I've heard officers complain when parents threaten to have their kids arrested if they don't behave. These kinds of threats set cops up to be bad guys and make kids afraid of them, rather than respect them. It will work the same with your own children.

Most little children are proud and happy to have a cop for a parent; they are the envy of many of their friends. This de-

pends on the community, of course, but young children generally have a positive regard for cops and associate them with
help and safety.

On the other hand, young children are very impressionable
and may assume their cop moms or dads are like TV cops—
always shooting and killing. A contributor to a booklet called
"You Know You're a Peace Officer's Wife When . . ." remembered a day when her young son came home from school crying.
One of his classmates told him that his daddy was going to get
killed because all police officers get killed. It was hard for this
mother to contain her own emotions and fears while she com-
forted her son, but she did. And then she and his father sat down
and talked to their child about death in general, about how well
trained his father was, and how being a police officer did not
mean he was going to die on the job.

Adolescents seem to be more at risk for public scrutiny from
their friends than are little children. Adolescence is a time when
kids are challenging adult authority, and it may be an especially
hard time for cops' kids. In some, but not all, teenage circles,
cops' kids may be challenged more than others to defy authority
and break the law in order to be part of the group. Or, they may
be stigmatized and ridiculed because their parent is a cop, and
cops are the very symbol of authority. Teens depend on their
friends a lot as they start to move toward independence from their
parents, and such pressures can create significant internal conflict
as a teenager feels his or her loyalties divided between friends and
family. A teenager's need for independence is normal and healthy,
but it can create undue anxiety for the parent who has intense
needs for safety control. Cops, in particular, need to guard against
overreacting to their teen's needs for autonomy.

Normal failings are not easily tolerated for police or preach-
ers' families. Police families often feel pressed to behave discreetly,
to have no conflicts, and to avoid any ostentatious behavior or
conspicuous consumption that would raise questions about cor-
ruption. The pressure is especially great on police families in
small, rural communities, where they know everyone and everyone knows them. It is hard to stand in the checkout line at the supermarket next to a person your mate has just arrested. It's even
harder when cops have to arrest someone they have known all

Tips for Dealing with Public Scrutiny

- Learn to deal in advance with intrusive or critical comments about police officers. Have a few prepared responses suitable for the occasion. Keep the tone humorous and light. (As a psychologist I often get pigeonholed at parties and inappropriately asked for advice about people I have never met, at which time I cheerfully tell those who are asking that I can't help them because I only deal with "easy cases." That usually gets a laugh and gets me off the hook.)

- Talk with your children about police work. Help them separate the myths from the realities. Give them as much information as they can handle. Monitor their TV watching so they don't get an overdose of death and danger from too many cop shows. Encourage them to go on ride-alongs, bring them into the station, and let them sit in a patrol car.

- Ride-alongs, by the way, are fabulous ways to understand what police work is all about. I encourage every cop's partner, friend, or family member to go on several ride-alongs. Chances are, you'll ride with someone other than your mate—this gives you the freedom to ask all kinds of questions and relieves your mate from having to show off.

- Let your children know when they are meeting your standards for good behavior and school performance. If they hear this regularly from you, they will be less vulnerable to other people's opinions about how they should act.

- Understand that you and your family have a right to privacy and aren't public property.

- Learn assertive communication skills so that you can end a conversation without starting a fight.

- Overreacting and defensiveness will usually add to the problem, not resolve it. Many people are interested in police work because it is exciting and stimulating. Take a minute to find out where people are coming from, and don't automatically assume they are being hostile. Police routinely underestimate the amount of admiration and respect their communities have for the work they do.

their lives. And while it doesn't happen all that often, sometimes your cop will be involved in an ongoing investigation of someone you know, and he or she can't tell you about it.

INJURIES

On-the-job injuries are a common occupational hazard. One of the reasons Danny was working so much overtime was to fill in for injured officers who were out on disability with broken shoulders, twisted knees, torn cartilage, and bad backs. There is little that is ergonomically correct about a police uniform or a police car. Cops get in and out of patrol cars dozens of times a day, wearing a minimum of 10 pounds of gear around their waists. More than once Danny's flashlight got twisted in his seat belt, and his baton got stuck in the steering wheel.

Some fitness trainers claim that officers who fail to stay in shape are at risk for injuring themselves. On the other hand, some of the folks Danny was filling in for had been fit athletes who were injured while training or competing.

Then there's the challenge of jumping fences and chasing people often half his age. Subduing reluctant suspects, *if* he caught them, was no easier. Danny was far from alone in getting beaten up. In 2004, about 16,500 officers were injured as a result of nearly 59,000 line-of-duty assaults.

SEPARATIONS AND LONG DEPLOYMENTS

Natural and man-made catastrophes have become all too frequent in the past decade. It is undeniable that when the next "big one" hits, whatever it is, your loved one will be running toward the disaster, not away from it. You may not see him or her for days.

In addition to responding to local calamities, police officers also participate in search and rescue or recovery efforts that may take them to other cities or states, occasionally even abroad. Sometimes they volunteer for these assignments; at other times they are deployed by their departments. The images of bravery and sacrifice at Ground Zero have been indelibly etched on our

---

Tips for Dealing with Injuries

- Keep fit: Officers and their families will benefit from a consistent, broad-based program of moderate activity that emphasizes flexibility, cardiovascular health, toned muscles, and relaxation skills.
- Create a recreation program that includes activities you can do as a couple or a family: hiking, biking, gardening, boating, dog walking, and so on.
- Pay attention to your stress level. Take stress management classes. Tension, especially muscle tension, may exacerbate injuries and prolong recovery.
- Review your defensive-tactics training on a regular basis.
- If you are injured, do what you can to avoid pushing yourself (or allowing yourself to be pushed) back to work prematurely.

---

collective consciousness, but there have been and will continue to be other catastrophic events—hopefully without such a massive loss of life—requiring police officers to spend prolonged amounts of time away from their families and their homes.

These long separations are hard on everyone in a family. One of the best ways police families can support each other through such trying times is to be prepared in advance, both mentally and in practical ways, for the separation and the reunion afterward.

Why reunions? Shouldn't homecoming be a happy time? Experience shows this isn't always so. The families of a local urban search and rescue team that went to Oklahoma City after the Alfred P. Murrah federal building was bombed by a terrorist took longer than expected to catch up with each other and reestablish intimacy. Rescuers were bombarded by the media and besieged by well-meaning community groups who wanted to reward their efforts and hear about their experiences. Some families complained that they learned more about the deployment by listening to their loved ones give interviews than they did by talking together. Children were sulky, distant, or clingy. Couples felt awkward with each other. Families fought over who had it worse during the deployment, and many spouses felt that no one had a clue about the effort it took for them to hold down the fort during separation. There were no award ceremonies for families.

Law enforcement families have to be tough, flexible, and independent. In 1999, my colleague Dr. Lorraine Greene and I got a grant from the National Institute for Justice to start a website for families, called policefamilies.com. As part of our grant, we conducted a survey of 420 police families. We had a novel approach: Rather than look at what goes wrong in police families, we wanted to find out what keeps them strong and resilient. What we found was that families who defined themselves as successful were flexible, were independent, had extended support systems, felt in control of their lives, and were supported by their law enforcement community. (See Bibliography, page 312, for a link to the full report.)

Tips for Dealing with Long Deployments and Reunions

- Become as self-sufficient as possible. Prepare your home and your family for emergencies. Learn how to do basic home repairs (for more information, see Chapters 8 and 13 and Resources).
- Get your loved one's department actively involved in supporting families who are left behind, or start a support network yourself. Ask the department to include families in disaster planning, prepare them for deployments, and help them cope with the after-action stress brought on by the media deluge and public clamor.
- Encourage the department to hold family briefings and/or set up a toll-free number for families to call for updates during deployment.
- Remind the department to include families in press releases and ceremonies honoring the returnees.
- Use electronic gadgets, such as cell phones and email, to stay in touch as the situation allows. Discuss in advance how and when you will do this.

(cont.)

(continued from previous page)

- Decide what decisions and family matters require input from both of you, which can be decided by the partner at home, and which should be postponed.
- Be sensitive to the challenges you each face. It's hard to be away from home and hard to be left behind. Be curious about each other's emotions and experiences. This will help you feel connected while you are apart.

At homecoming:

- Be patient. Keep your expectations realistic. It takes time to get reacquainted and for life to return to normal.
- Make time to talk individually and as a family. Young children, especially, need time to warm up to a parent who has been absent. All children will want to talk about what has happened to them during their parents' absence.
- Avoid scheduling too many things; your officer needs rest. After an intense experience, it takes time to return to the normal pace of life. Understand that some officers may alternate between wanting to talk and not wanting to talk, especially if they're tired and still processing what happened during deployment.
- If you've changed the way you normally make decisions or discipline the kids during deployment, discuss these changes with your mate and try to meet each other halfway. Try to be open-minded and avoid criticizing each other for changes made while you were apart.
- Reread the tips for dealing with long hours and shift work in this chapter; the section Kids and Trauma, dealing with separations, in Chapter 8; and the tip section in Chapter 13, "Cop Couples."

CHAPTER 2

THE POLICE OFFICER'S PARADOX

To function effectively in our job, you must annihilate, smother, and suppress normal emotions like fear, anger, revulsion, and even compassion. To do otherwise is to invite overwhelming doubt or hesitancy when decisive action is required. The penalty for your achieved competence is a mind set that might as well be a foreign language to your social contemporaries. We are . . . victims of our own success. When these same normal and appropriate emotions . . . surface in personal relationships, we automatically shut down and wonder why, over time, that the people we care about the most complain that we are aloof, cold, and uncommunicative.
—Ret. Captain Al Benner, PhD

It is a paradox that the same work habits that make a good cop can be hazardous to being a good mate and parent. Marvin is a case in point. He policed his family the way he worked the streets. He was highly critical of his wife and children and overcontrolling of his household. He had grown fearful and suspicious during his years on the job, and consequently, he rarely took his family on vacation because he was uncomfortable in unfamiliar places. His concerns for order were so excessive that he supervised ordinary household tasks like dishwashing and watering the yard. No one in his family dared argue or contradict him. The price he paid for this level of control was an almost total loss of intimacy, spontaneity, and positive regard from his wife and children, who were angry or frightened of him most of the time.

Marvin had to unlearn what he had learned so well from the academy and afterward. He had to recognize that hypervigilance, emotional control, a command presence, and a skeptical, if not outright suspicious, attitude toward others are professional habits to be left at work.

Anna, his wife, had things to learn as well. Although she was a competent, well-paid professional, she had to learn to ask for what she needed and insist on getting it. She was depressed from years of believing she was obligated to take a back seat to Marvin—something she had learned from her own mother, who had subjugated herself to Anna's father, a man even more stern and domineering than Marvin.

Anna had to give herself permission to take time for herself and not feel guilty for needing help with the family. She was so angry with Marvin, she paid little attention to him as a person beyond blindly acceding to his demands in order to get him off her back. Once Anna found the courage to tell Marvin how unhappy she was and find ways to get her own needs met, their relationship warmed considerably. They were committed to marriage and family, and at no time did either seriously consider divorce. Rather, they passively accepted the belief that their lives together would always be filled with unexpressed resentments and longings.

Obviously, there was a lot more influencing Marvin and Anna's relationship than hazardous work habits. Both had negative role models from their families of origin, and both were influenced by cultural stereotypes of male and female behavior. Finding their way out of this unhappy relationship to a more balanced partnership would require both their efforts. Looking at the hazardous habits Marvin had acquired at work and how these were affecting the family was a good place to start.

EMOTIONAL CONTROL

From the beginning, cops are taught to maintain an occupational persona: a "public face" that makes them always appear to be in control, on top of things, knowledgeable, and unafraid. In fact, much of the stress of police work is a result of trying to hide the strain and pressure of the job. Police work is emotional labor. Officers are required to control their own emotions, as well as the emotional reactions of others—getting civilians to calm down, comply with orders, submit to authority, and so on. Good street officers cannot afford to give anything away to suspects by letting their feelings show. They can't tell a child molester that they are repulsed by his actions if they expect to get a confession. They can't weep during a death notification, even if they want to, because their presence should stabilize the crisis. They can't let their anger out when they are hit, spat on, or humiliated. In fact, cops rarely show sadness, fear, or uncertainty in front of each other because they dread losing support and respect. Since police officers depend on one another for safety, mutual support is crucial to their well-being.

For example, let's discuss what happened to Dick, who had half-empty conversations about something important that occurred to him. He could share part of the story at work and part of the story at home, but he had to keep the whole story to himself. Dick was pursuing a recklessly driven vehicle through downtown streets during rush hour. It was a perilous chase as the errant driver hit one car after another while Dick followed helplessly behind, unable to safely make a move. Finally, he was able to block the other car and bring it to a stop. The driver leapt from the vehicle in a terribly agitated state, and Dick had to use force to subdue him. The driver, who was sobbing and hysterical, was drunk and in need of hospitalization. On the way to the hospital, the driver identified himself as a disabled police officer.

Back at the station, Dick discussed the incident with other cops, telling them about the exhilaration of the pursuit but hiding the sorrow he felt for the driver. At home, he shared the sorrow, but he couldn't talk about the dangerous yet exhilarating chase because he didn't want to worry his wife.

Questions whirled in his head: "Is this job damaging me too?" "Is it aging me?" "What if I can't top this?" "What if I get bored?" These were healthy, normal questions. But, because Dick felt he needed to maintain control and not show worry or empathy, he isolated himself and didn't have the benefit of discussing all of his concerns with the people he most trusted.

In the beginning, emotional control may feel like acting. After a while, it becomes a habit an officer cannot turn on and off at will. This is a *big* dilemma: Officers are rewarded for maintaining emotional distance in the performance of their duties and punished for doing so in their personal relationships, where this same emotional control causes them to hurt and alienate those they love and need.

Officers exert emotional control, not because they don't have feelings, but because they may have defended themselves so well against their feelings that they have blunted their ability to recognize sensibilities in themselves or in others or to express any but the most potent emotions. And then they may reserve these most potent emotions for special circumstances, such as sporting events or police funerals.

Your officer may want or need to talk about something but may hesitate to do so for fear of losing control. Rather than reliving the incident, he or she may decide it's safer not to talk at all and may create a convenient fiction as justification: "My wife doesn't want to hear this; she won't understand, and anyhow, I don't want to worry her."

Officers have been indoctrinated to keep a lid on their feelings. They are warned repeatedly that losing control can jeopardize their safety *and* their career. Because they have stifled so much emotion, they fear that letting out just a little may start a flood that can't be stopped.

Rather than risk being emotionally swamped, some officers may avoid an uncomfortable topic by drowning their sorrows in liquor. Or they may overfocus on someone else—a spouse, a child, or an administrator—instead of looking at their own feelings. Or they may distance themselves from the family—a common tactic among men, in particular.

I worked with Phil for a long time after he had shot and killed a suspected burglar. Week after week he told me in a calm, controlled manner how much this event had disrupted his life and caused him monumental psychic pain. *What* he was talking about and *how* he was talking about it didn't jibe. One day I commented on the incongruity of how he presented himself. He burst into tears and cried for a long time, until his eyes swelled up and he was exhausted by the effort of releasing what must have felt like a tidal wave of emotion. It was the turning point in his recovery.

Because officers are taught to control their emotions in the face of utter chaos, their families may have to work hard to get their attention, which can breed anger and hysteria. By the same token, officers are so adept at looking for danger signals, they may miss the expression of more subtle emotions. For example, cops are trained to keep their eyes on a suspect's hands, not on his or her face, because if they are going to get hurt, the weapon will be in the suspect's hands, not on his or her head. Years of this kind of training compromise an officer's sensitivity to other forms of nonverbal expression that make up a large part of how we communicate with each other.

Another reason officers feel a need to exert control over their emotions is because they see so much distress and despair. Testifying about police family stress before Congress, police psychologist Dr. Ellen Scrivner said that the average officer will see more human tragedy in the first three years of his or her career than the average person sees in a lifetime. As a result of seeing so much despair, cops develop "compassion fatigue." They are wise to protect themselves from this steady diet of human tragedy, no question. What is problematic is that they protect themselves by overcontrolling their normal reactions and distancing themselves from their emotions. Retired FBI agent Jim Reese says, "We in law enforcement have become very adept at turning our emotions off. It is the 'on switch' that many of us cannot find."

Feelings are the deepest part of us. We cannot ask for what we need or make decisions on our own behalf unless we have access to the depth of our feelings. Intimacy occurs between people who are able to reveal their most private thoughts and emotions to each other. To do so requires risk and the willingness to feel vulnerable and exposed. There is an inherent paradox here. *You have to lose control in order to gain it.* It is hard to take risks without having a safe place to do so. Ideally, the best safe place is the circle of family and friends.

CYNICISM AND OVERPROTECTIVENESS

There are two other dimensions related to emotional control that affect friends and families. One is the officer's efforts to protect his or her family from the gritty realities of life. The other is cynicism, the belief that most human behavior is motivated by selfishness. A cynic expects nothing good from people and is therefore rarely disappointed. In an indirect way, cynical cops are trying to protect both themselves and the people they love from being hurt or becoming victims.

Cynicism results from prolonged exposure to the worst in people's behavior—cops see a lot of that. No one calls a cop when he or she is having a good day. People lie to cops about everything: who they are, what they have been doing, what their name is, and so on. Even ordinarily law-abiding citizens are known to bend the truth about their driving habits. It takes only a few disappointments for an idealistic young officer to build a self-protective wall of cynicism against being made to look foolish or feel naive. There is so much cynicism in police work that the cynical officer easily finds like-minded company to reinforce his or her position.

Sid was very cynical. As far as he was concerned, every boy who showed up to date his daughter was no good. Maybe every father feels protective toward his teenage daughter, or perhaps Sid is remembering his own teenage behavior. Sid was extreme in his reactions, occasionally checking his daughter's dates for criminal history, which was against department regulations. He made no effort to get to know any of them or even engage them in conversation. Whenever his wife or daughter complained about his behavior, he dismissed them by pulling rank—he, after all, was a cop and knew more about people's motives than they did because they were naive and easily fooled. Needless to say, it didn't take long before his daughter started meeting her dates someplace else, and Sid lost the very control he was trying to exert. He lost his daughter's confidence and respect, as well.

Some officers are so eager to keep their home a sanctuary that they create barriers rather than shift gears between home and work. They become overprotective, discussing little if anything about their life away from home. Their fears and anxieties for the family's safety may be so extreme that they overrestrict the family's activities and do not permit family members to have a normal range of motion in the world or to choose for themselves what friends they will have and what activities they will pursue.

When cops try to protect their families from the realities of life, they must engage in some deception about how successful or content they are at work. One officer, who battled continuously with his wife over neatness and cleanliness, insightfully observed that he had the luxury of keeping all his mistakes and failures to himself, whereas his wife was fair game for criticism because everything she did or didn't do at home was out in the open.

It is popular to talk these days about being in denial. Overprotective officers have just the opposite problem: They cannot turn off their concerns and worries. They develop a kind of tunnel vision, tending to isolate themselves from others and associate only with other cops; therefore, they have a limited reality check on the universe. They come to believe that their world of work is a mirror of the world at large. If and when you try to suggest a different perspective, you may be told you don't know what you are talking about because you aren't a cop. This is both hurtful and inaccurate, but it may be exactly how the overprotective and cynical cop sees things.

To say the least, it is frustrating to live with an officer who cannot let his or her guard down, who is remote, cynical, or overprotective. If this is happening in your relationship, you may feel alienated and lonely. You may not know what to do; you may withdraw, distance yourself, and pretend that you don't care. Like the officer, you may begin using emotional control as a defense against strong feelings of rejection, alienation, isolation, and loneliness. Or you may begin to overfunction, to pursue your officer in an attempt to get him or her to open up. This is a common dance between men and women—he distances and she pursues. It is a strategy that rarely works, although it is understandable that you would want to make a connection with the person you love if you feel that he or she is emotionally distant.

CHAINED TO THE CHAIN OF COMMAND

Cops probably spend as much time controlling others as they do controlling themselves. As a matter of fact, most activities in police work have to do with controlling something or someone: traffic control, crowd control, crime control, budget control, overtime control, and so on.

Police agencies are paramilitary organizations structured according to rank. Power and authority are distributed along a chain of command. Some people protest that this simple organizational structure is outdated and no longer effective. But in the main, cops are comfortable with the clarity and simplicity of the paramilitary system because it works well in emergencies when someone needs to be in charge. Cops are comfortable with giving orders and taking them, and they accept this as a norm of their profession.

An officer who has been trained to give and receive orders without argument may expect compliance at home and react poorly to not being able to get it. The odds, of course, are against being able to control family members as though they were suspects, law breakers, or people who need to be ordered about. Most families won't, and shouldn't, accept being treated in this way.

Jackie's experience is a good example of how and when you can put your foot down. When Jackie's husband, Lester, was promoted, they were both overjoyed. His success was a long time in coming, and Jackie felt she had earned this promotion too because she had sacrificed a lot so that Lester could put in the extra time and energy required to climb this high up the ladder. She was therefore shocked and hurt when Lester began acting "too big for his britches." He had a noticeable attitude change and started demanding, rather than asking, for things at home. Jackie tolerated his attitude for a few weeks, and when it didn't change, she confronted him and reminded him that she, more than anyone, knew he put his pants on one leg at a time. She told him to leave his gold bars behind when he came home. She expected to be treated with respect and not taken for granted. Specifically, she requested he say "please" and "thank you" when he asked for her help.

When cops experience family problems, or know that the people they love are troubled, they may expect to be able to solve those problems in the same way they solve problems at work. They may feel frustrated and ashamed at their inability to do so and see it instead as a lack of compliance—if you would do as they say, you'd be happier or get along better.

The failure to get compliance raises an officer's anxiety because he or she has been trained from the start to believe that a noncompliant suspect constitutes a threat to officer safety. Furthermore, when cops themselves are noncompliant, they risk getting disciplined or jeopardize their chances for promotion.

Ordering people about is especially hard on adolescent children who are normally rebellious and challenging as a part of their maturing. Overinterpreting their rebellious activity or, worse still, confusing it with a threat to physical safety can cause unnecessary problems.

Because cops do so much catastrophizing—expecting the worst possible outcome at all times—they are apt to overreact to children's noncompliance. One cop told me he was fingerprinting objects in his house in order to solve the mystery of which of his children had taken some money. I thought there were other, less policelike ways of getting to the bottom of the matter. His children needed a father, not a house cop. They also needed to learn ways to ask for what they needed, rather than steal it, and to tolerate the disappointment they felt if they didn't get what they wanted. What I think they learned instead was how not to get caught the next time.

There is little hope a child will confide in a parent who takes an investigative rather than understanding approach toward problem solving. Treat a child as a suspect often enough, and that child may begin to act like a criminal.

Consider Pete, who was playing miniature golf with his family. The person in front of him was not playing fast enough to suit Pete, a speedy, type A person. He first asked the man to play faster; then he asked him to move aside and let Pete and his family pass. When the man didn't respond to this request, Pete screamed at him, grabbed him by the shirt, and threw him aside. The manager threw Pete and his family out, the golf game was ruined, and Pete's kids learned that the way to handle a problem was through intimidation and muscle.

Command presence is designed to be intimidating and best left in the work locker. It is nearly impossible for friends and family to have a relaxed, mutual conversation with someone trained in interrogation skills, covered with image armor, and filled with excessive certainty about his or her own views and opinions.

I often have to gear up to deal with the combative conversational style of many cops I work with. I have to remind myself that humor is the way some cops express affection before I remind them that there are other ways to reveal their fondness for someone. There are times when I am exhilarated by engaging in linguistic combat, or I wouldn't be in this business. But there are other days when I am tired or preoccupied, and this challenging style feels irritating and adolescent—the humor stings more than it salves.

I have a friend who is a librarian and is married to an attorney who is highly verbal and used to duking it out in court with equally verbal adversaries. She, true to her profession, is quiet, introspective, and service oriented. She is not comfortable with conflict. He runs circles around her verbally, which makes her feel powerless and frustrated at the inequity in their verbal skills. When she asserts herself, it costs her a great deal emotionally: She feels exhausted and self-doubting, as if she has turned into a bitch or a nag.

Her husband, on the other hand, feels exhilarated by confrontation. He is energized by the challenge and by the sound of his own arguments and verbal acumen. However, he is discomforted by feeling he has steamrolled over his wife, whom he truly adores, and wishes that his natural verbal energy and forceful personality were not so overwhelming to her. He has a hard time slowing down and is often repentant over things he has said in the heat of debate.

My friend has had to learn to be more assertive in order to level the playing field with her husband. She has acquired a set of competencies—tools that she uses to hold her own without becoming an in-your-face, strident, confrontational person. She learned to do the following by reading and taking a class in assertiveness at her local community college.

- Stand up for your rights.
- Express your opinions.
- Offer constructive criticism.
- Initiate conversations.
- End conversations.
- Reject unreasonable criticism or demands.
- Disagree with the opinions of others.
- Make your needs and wishes known.

- Accept and give compliments.
- Seek out friends.
- Make suggestions.
- Say no when appropriate.
- Ask for information.
- Tell others about yourself.

There are many excellent books on the subject of assertiveness (see Recommended Reading in the Resources section), and many community colleges offer classes in assertiveness training. Being assertive is a valuable competency in dealing with life in general and, in particular, with any cops you know who are badge-heavy and authoritarian.

HYPERVIGILANCE

Steve called me at home on a Sunday morning. He had had two heart attack scares for which there was no medical basis. He thought he was going crazy. He couldn't sit still; he couldn't eat or do anything but pace. Nothing was wrong with him medically, but still he couldn't lose the feeling of doom that hovered over him.

Steve was suffering from panic attacks, and his panic attacks represented the extreme outcome of uncontrolled hypervigilance. Not everyone who experiences hypervigilance winds up with panic attacks, but nearly everyone who works as a cop experiences some hypervigilance.

Hypervigilance is a hazardous habit that alters the way cops interact with their environment. It is a hard habit to break because it is so highly reinforced. From day one, cops are taught to see nearly everything in their environment as potentially life threatening and dangerous. They are urged, warned, required, and rewarded for developing a habit of scanning the environment for cues to danger. They are taught that their survival and the survival of others depend on their ability to interpret most of their environment as potentially lethal. In other words, they learn to look around and ask "what if" questions about everything.

At some point, hypervigilance appears to actually change something in a part of the neurological system that is responsible for scanning the environment for threats. Average citizens don't experience these changes because we have not been coaxed into and rewarded for questioning the threat potential of every thing or every person we see.

This scanning behavior becomes so finely tuned that even mild danger alerts the officer's autonomic nervous system. The cop experiences this as a buzz: a general sense of aliveness, high energy, vitality, and alertness. This state of physiological elevation becomes its own reward, like a runner's high. Dr. Kevin Gilmartin, retired sheriff's deputy, thinks this is what cops mean when they talk about police work getting into their blood or about becoming addicted to their own adrenalin. Over time, officers may begin to "overinterpret" danger signals and lose the ability to distinguish between situations that are potentially lethal and those that are not: PTA meetings, a night at the movies, a drive in the country, a meal in a restaurant, and a party can all become potentially dangerous events in which the officer spends more time figuring out other people's motives and secret intentions than interacting or relaxing. I've heard too many tales of mates and children being left on the sidewalk, caught up in vehicle pursuits, stranded in restaurants, abandoned in movie theaters, and stuck in shopping malls when what started out as a normal family outing turned into police work. (This may not always be the result of hypervigilance since many departments require officers to carry weapons 24 hours a day and be prepared to take action when needed. This policy is not family friendly.)

Police officers are caught in a bind, just like doctors. Both hold positions of public trust and are trained to respond to emergencies. Society demands that they get involved, and they expect it of themselves as well. The problem arises when cops become so hypervigilant that they actually search for an opportunity to get involved in an emergency because they need that hit of adrenalin to avoid feeling depressed or listless. Or they develop a sense of superiority to anyone—including their family members—who doesn't share their alarmist point of view.

Leon's story illustrates the bind cops are in. Leon and his 10-year-old son, Rick, were on vacation together in a motel. Their time together was precious to both of them. Looking out the window, Leon spotted what appeared to be a bad guy with a gun in a car in the parking lot. He immediately went into action. He closed the blinds to his window and ordered his son to go into the bathroom and lie down in the bathtub in case there was gunfire. He watched the man walk up to the motel and then walk away after knocking on a few doors and getting no response.

Leon debated whether or not to call the local police with a description. The man with the gun might have been an undercover cop. Or he might not have been, in which case Leon worried that an unsuspecting cop might pull this guy over and get shot. On the other hand, he was concerned that if he called the police, he would sacrifice the afternoon by giving statements. He opted to take his son on their planned hike, but he continued to worry about his choice and second-guessed his decision not to call.

Is this hypervigilance? Excessive responsibility? The weight of the badge? The dilemma of a man of integrity whose roles as both father and police officer were in conflict? I think this case may be a combination of all four, which underscores just how complicated this policing business is.

The behavior of a hypervigilant officer can be like a roller coaster because adrenalin, like other drugs, has a rebound effect: As a person "comes down" from the drug, he or she experiences an effect directly opposite to the one originally craved.

Let's return to Steve who had panic attacks. After a day of police work he would return home so exhausted that he would drop into a state of vegetation in front of the TV set, able only to channel-surf. He backed off from family activities so often that his wife, Ginger, stopped asking him along because she and the kids didn't want to risk further rejection.

When Steve went on a family vacation, he would ruminate about possible dangers. If he was taking his kids boating for the day, he imagined the boat turning over and saw himself diving into the murky water, searching desperately for his kids. He could actually feel the water and experience his utter panic. His blood pressure increased, his breathing became shallow and rapid, his heart rate quickened, and he experienced spurts of adrenalin. The same panic occurred at work. It became Steve's habit to expect the worst possible outcome on every call. His mental preparation went far beyond getting ready for the possibility of significant violence to actually inventing the disturbance and playing the whole thing out in his head, just as if it were a movie. Even after successfully and peacefully handling an incident, he would replay it in his head several times with different, more violent outcomes.

At home, Steve could only rouse himself from his post-hypervigilant stupor by novelty buying. Whenever he felt listless and depressed, he went to the local electronics store or tool shop and bought another gadget. There were two beneficiaries of this habit: his credit card company and his neighbors, who knew they could borrow anything they needed from Steve. If he didn't have it, he would buy it.

Tips for Dealing with Hazardous Work Habits

- Shift gears. Encourage your officer to enter a new mindset before returning home: Jogging, playing sports, or working out will help refocus the mind, relax the body, and provide an outlet for the accumulated tensions of the day. Exercise has many stress-reducing and health-promoting benefits. Even moderate exercise, like walking or gardening, is helpful in decontaminating the adrenalin produced by hypervigilance.
- Keep your nonpolice friends even though scheduling makes this difficult. If the burden of setting up a social calendar falls on you, so will the benefits. You need to be part of the community at large in order to avoid becoming isolated. When you have friends outside the department, you can confide in them without worrying about contributing to departmental gossip. Social support is a very positive and productive way to cope with stress.
- Stay involved with a variety of people and activities: sports events, school events, church, the arts, volunteer work, and community festivities. Cops and their families need to interact in a positive way with good, productive people of all ages, races, and professions or they forget such people exist.
(cont.)

(continued from previous page)

- In social situations, don't overfunction for your spouse or cover for his or her cynicism. If your mate makes a cynical remark, don't feel guilty by association. You'll be judged for yourself.
- Learn and practice good time-management skills (see Recommended Reading). Dr. Gilmartin suggests that scheduling dates and sticking to those commitments work better than doing things when "you feel like it." Hypervigilant cops are so emotionally exhausted by work that they rarely feel like doing anything but channel surfing or restimulating their autonomic nervous systems. Schedule family activities before hitting the remote control. Meet your officer after work and go from there. Positive experiences will tend to be self-reinforcing.

CHAPTER 3

GROWING OLD IN A YOUNG PERSON'S PROFESSION

How Officers Change with Time

> I was rushing to get to work when my 16-year-old daughter called to me, "Hey, Robocop. Can you file a missing person's report for me?" My heart stopped. I thought one of her friends had run away. "Who's missing?" I asked. "My mother," she answered.
> —CHIEF LILLIE LEONARDI

Looking forward may be the best insurance we have against being blind-sided by the unexpected. This is especially true in love and in police work, when, in the beginning, emotions run so high and are so gratifying that it is hard to think things will ever change or to prepare ourselves for changes we can't imagine.

Long-term police careers and long-lived marriages in general seem to follow a U-shaped course, with satisfaction declining and then increasing in incremental phases. Many psychologists and cops agree about this, though we differ slightly on the specifics. These are not important differences because this is a map, not a timetable. Everyone will chart his or her course differently.

FALLING IN LOVE WITH THE JOB: THE APPLICANT PHASE

Do people who consider policing as a career have anything in common? Is there such a thing as a typical police personality?

43

This is a hotly debated issue. For my money, no one really knows. Even the question "What kind of person makes a good police officer?" has not been answered except in the most general terms: someone who is intelligent, emotionally stable, and can take decisive action quickly and in proportion to the situation at hand.

Psychologists who screen prospective officers are the first to admit that they are more effective at screening people out than predicting who will make a good police officer and why. Pre-employment screening gives us only a snapshot of the entry-level police officer. The picture we get after the wear and tear of the work itself may be very different.

In general, people who consider policing as a career are community-minded and action-oriented. They are comfortable giving and taking orders and are willing to be decisive and visible. They often have high security needs and, at the same time, require variety and stimulation and dislike being confined to an office. They take pride in their work and are willing to conform to group norms. They value control, both in themselves and in their environment, which is important because they often arrive on the scene when control is lost. They are honest, well adjusted, extroverted, independent, assertive, and have an average or above-average IQ. They may be, or become, emotionally guarded and can suppress their feelings while under stress. They are often funny and can use wit and humor as a tool, a weapon, or a way to camouflage feelings. They are resistant to change and rely on standard procedures to do their work. They have an eye for detail. They value predictability. They are protection-oriented and may have assumed the role of protector or rescuer in their families as they were growing up. They are perfectionistic and have high standards for themselves and others. They are great in a crisis and rate high on mental stability.

Applying for a police position is a strenuous, time-consuming endeavor. By the time applicants successfully pass all the requirements—application forms, written testing, interviews, role playing, background investigation, medical and psychological examinations, and so forth—they feel like specially chosen members of an elite club of superior people. If applicants were merely interested in the job before, during the process it has become such a prize that they are usually *in love* with the idea of being a cop by the time they are hired. Candidates deserve to be proud of their persistence and abilities: Barely two out of 100 police applicants are successful in getting the job.

AT THE ACADEMY AND ON PROBATION

Rookies are eager suitors. Having won the job, they now have to hold onto it and prove their worth. They have two tasks to accomplish: fitting in and being competent.

New officers are at the beginning of a prestigious career that brings responsibility, challenge, and opportunity, as well as financial security. For most, the gratification of being part of this accomplished group of professionals far exceeds, for now, the costs of conforming to the group.

Without realizing it, the rookie officer is taking on a new identity as much as he or she is beginning a new career. Hardly anyone considers this just a job. Excitement is high; anxiety is up. Bonding with fellow rookies for practical help and social support eases the anxiety about getting through. Depending on coworkers will become a lifelong habit, one that is considered critical to survival in the job and on the street.

At home, you are much the same as any family or friend with a buddy in graduate or medical school. Your cop doesn't have as much time for you as he or she did before. He will be tired, physically and mentally. She will feel anxious and guilty about taking time away from her studies even when a break would do her good. He or she will seem consumed with studying and more interested in police work than in you or anything else. You may have to remind your cop that, while you understand these are unusual times and you will be flexible, it isn't acceptable to you to be totally left out or neglected.

This is a temporary state: Concern about succeeding is intense because the stakes are high. Rookies have no job security and won't until probation is over. They do get support since most departments have a considerable financial investment in new officers and work hard to help them be successful.

Edward's experience is typical of the kind of pressure cooker officers are in during field training. Edward appeared in my office

45

on the verge of tears. He was doing acceptable work in the field training program, but he would occasionally make minor errors and receive lower than acceptable ratings. He reacted to these low ratings as if each was a prelude to termination.

One of the ways he tried to cope with his anxiety was to second-guess his field training officer (FTO). That made his work harder because he now had to think for himself at the same time he was trying to read her mind—an impossible task that interfered with concentrating on his driving and what was happening around him.

At home, he was having trouble sleeping, and he ignored his wife and small child. When his wife complained about this, he overreacted. It was as though he could do nothing right at work and now nothing right at home. He displaced his frustration onto his wife, Meg, and blew up when she told him how overwhelmed and lonely she felt at home all day with their infant son. Needless to say, that made matters worse, and Edward was in a very bad mood when he reported for work the next day. After talking with him, we agreed he needed counseling on two fronts, at home and at work. His FTO and I talked about his performance, and she assured him that he was not doing as poorly as he imagined.

At home, Edward apologized to Meg, and they talked about what was going on for both of them. Edward encouraged Meg to spend more time with friends and to join a gym that had childcare facilities, so she wasn't stuck at home all day. They began to talk about her returning to work, at least part time, as much for the social interaction as the needed income. Edward agreed to take one morning of his days off to be with his child, in exchange for which his wife agreed to help quiz him on the penal code. They also made plans to drive around the city where Edward worked: This killed several birds with one stone, so to speak: They were able to spend time together; Edward got to work on learning his way around the city, something he needed to improve; and Meg got to see the community where Edward was working.

Officers in training often feel they are not doing much right and doubt their ability to absorb the mountain of information they need to know. There's a lot families can do to help. Worry can be contagious: Try to be reassuring and encouraging, but don't get caught up in the doubt. Do what you are comfortable doing to get involved. Learn as much as you want about what's happening and what your cop is studying. Attend academy events held for the family. Go on ride-alongs at the police department—you'll learn a lot. At the same time, stick to your own schedule and don't neglect your obligations. Negotiate spending enough time together every week so that *each* of you can talk about what's going on in your life. Try to engage in some lighthearted, distracting activities together, like hiking.

If at all possible, don't make any large purchases that will create big bills until after probation—in other words, don't count your chickens before they hatch. Debt adds greatly to the anxiety and pressure. The academy and the field training program are places to learn, but they are also secondary levels of screening, and a certain percentage of officers—some 15 to 25%—will not successfully complete the program or will recognize that they have chosen the wrong career and leave. Although those who leave or are terminated often regard themselves as failures, I think it is a painful but lucky break to discover early on that a person doesn't like or is unsuited to this career. It is much harder to shake those "golden handcuffs" and leave the job later on.

As a matter of fact, if it were up to me, I would structure a police career in five-year increments and make it easier for officers to use their valuable police training as a steppingstone to another career. I recognize this is a controversial suggestion. These days, qualified applicants are hard to find, and losing experienced officers can affect both the efficiency and safety of those left behind. On the other hand, the organization recovers its initial investment in the individual officer in about five years, nearly the same time he or she is beginning to confront some of the unpleasant realities of the job.

PHASE ONE: THE HONEYMOON

The early years following training are the most "heady" and "delicious" of an officer's career. Retired Police Chief Karel Swanson of Walnut Creek, California, describes this time as almost utter intoxication, novelty in its purest form: "Every encounter is a chance to encourage, manipulate, intimidate, confront, or impress others." The learning curve is high, and each day brings a new opportunity to test oneself and perform in a way never thought possible. Your officer is carrying levels of responsibility and authority that probably exceed anything he or she has experienced before. Officers feel energized and truly alive. They are exposed to people and events they never before dreamed of. Some of these experiences may be frightening, revolting, or disturbing, but the novelty is what counts most. Officers now have license to enter worlds that were previously forbidden to them, and some are drawn to these shadowy sides of life in the way that circus goers are drawn to sideshows.

New officers feel invincible, as though they are fulfilling a kind of hero role—protector; rescuer; powerful, brave defender of justice. They are consumed with police work and eager to discuss shop, especially with other cops on their squad. At this point, the rookie's enthusiasm for work obscures any disadvantages of the job, and the officer thinks that he or she can happily do this forever! Some psychologists think this early intoxication only sows the seeds for a hard fall into disillusionment.

The other day, I stopped a new solo officer on his way out of the police garage to ask him how things were going now that he was out of the field training program. He had this huge grin on his face. "I can't believe they pay me to do this job" he said, as though he had gotten away with something. I shared this with a veteran officer, also on his way out of the garage, and we agreed, feeling sad and wise at the same time: In a few years, if this officer was true to form, he would not only feel he deserved every penny he earned but would also complain that he wasn't being paid enough.

Although the honeymoon phase may be the "most delicious" of a cop's career, it is also stressful because it is filled with change, challenge, and a constant measuring up against the demands of the job. Rookies are learning to deal with intense emotions as they are exposed to things most of us will never see. Some develop a protective coating of aloofness and superrationality referred to as the John or Jayne Wayne syndrome.

This phase is tough on families. You may feel as if you are playing second fiddle to the job. You may sense that you and your concerns have been relegated to the background, and you're expected to keep your problems to yourself and not burden your spouse. You may feel as if things are backward, that you exist to support the job instead of the other way around. You may wonder what happened to the person you once knew.

Hollis was like this as a rookie. Here he was, at 22 years of age, vested with more power than most people have in a lifetime. He ate, slept, and dreamt about police work. He literally vibrated with anticipation during briefings. He got to work early and stayed late. He was busy impressing his coworkers and his supervisors with his enthusiasm; and, in fact, he didn't have to manufacture this, because he was jazzed beyond belief about police work.

After work, all he wanted to do was debrief with his buddies. Going home to the roommates he'd had since college, who were engineers and software designers, was too boring: All they did was talk about computers and sports. He used to like sports, but now work was his sport. When he did get home, he was critical and thought he could handle the domestic chores more efficiently than his roommates. He had an opinion on everything, including the evening news and all the cop shows.

When they went out for a pizza, he took his gun and made so many observations about criminal activity on the street that it cast a negative pall on the evening. For a while, his roommates were eager to hear about his work, but they soon got tired of pulling his share of the load because he was too busy—which soon came to mean too important—to pitch in. They also complained to each other that their accomplishments and their problems paled in comparison to Hollis's. They stopped telling him anything personal, and Hollis soon moved out of their apartment and in with some police officers.

It's important to start now to problem-solve with your mate or your friend. This is preventive medicine to stop communication problems before they start. Try not to "gunnysack" your resentments: Don't let them stack up until you blow up or until there is such a mountain of resentments that you can't dig yourself out. As things come up, communicate them to your mate in a timely fashion. Ann Coughlin, Sharon Hern, and Judy Ard, all police spouses, recommend starting in the first year to bargain hard for your relationship. It is wise—though not always possible—to do so in a calm, thoughtful manner rather than when you are upset or angry.

For example, Karen was frequently late coming home from work, which angered and frightened her husband, Manny, who often imagined the worst. Manny was frustrated: He didn't know if he should eat dinner or wait for Karen because she could be anywhere from 30 minutes to three hours late.

When Manny raised this issue with Karen, he was calm. He said this was a major concern because it happened regularly. He understood that Karen's work was unpredictable and that Karen didn't always have control over the unpredictability, but he thought she could always get to a phone within a reasonable time. He was straightforward and didn't overdramatize her behavior; for example, he didn't assume her lateness meant she didn't care about him or the family.

Karen, however, resented his suggestion. She told Manny she felt as though he was her father and that she didn't have to "report in" and "ask permission." Manny stuck to his ground and said it was unacceptable for him to be left hanging. He valued his time with Karen and wanted to wait for her, providing he knew how long that would be. Manny emphasized that he was not trying to control Karen's life but to control his own. Karen finally revealed that she was afraid of being humiliated in front of the "guys," who would tease her for having to tell her husband where she was. She felt this would make her look foolish—if she couldn't stand up to her husband, how could she confront the bad guys?

Manny didn't budge from his bottom line. He told Karen that handling the taunts of her shift mates was her concern, and he wasn't playing second fiddle to her need for their approval. He offered to help Karen figure out a snappy, lighthearted response to their teasing, but he clearly said that he expected her allegiance to be to him first.

The next time Karen was delayed and telephoned home, she did get teased. She responded by telling the guys that they were afraid to tell their "mommies" they would be late, that she was a grown up and was taking responsibility for managing her marriage. Some of the guys got the hint and called their wives; some of them didn't. But Karen had broken the ice, and she and Manny eliminated a nagging source of resentment.

Manny and Karen solved this issue in a straightforward way, with little upset. They also made a symbolic statement about the relative value of work and family. Most important, they established a pattern of action that dictated when one of us has a problem, we all do—and we all participate in solving it. Manny complained, but he hung in there to help Karen figure out how to do her part. Neither abandoned the other or rejected responsibility.

These kinds of habits and values get seeded in a family early on. Frequently, rookie officers are starting new families at the same time as they are starting new careers. This is a lot to deal with. I cannot emphasize enough the importance of keeping the channels of communication open and learning how to settle disputes, make decisions, and move ahead before things pile up. Managing a family is like managing an organization. Love isn't enough.

PHASE TWO: SETTLING DOWN

You've survived the rookie years. Your officer is competent and confident in his or her street skills. The job is still interesting, but the novelty has started to wear thin, and some of the thrill is gone. You may see some telltale signs of cynicism.

The rescue fantasies that he or she had in the academy have been tempered with a more realistic appraisal of the limits of police work and police officers. Your cop has learned to be satisfied with a few successes. Fantasies about the job itself have been replaced with a more realistic acceptance of the boring and frustrating parts: the mountains of paperwork, the influence of politics, the flaws in the judicial system, and the relentless hammering of the media. Most illusions about the basic goodness of human beings have been flattened into a persistent skepticism. Only the most innocent of victims—children or old people—merit much compassion.

Your officer may start looking around for new ways to be stimulated and challenged in order to regain that early sense of thrill that was so emotionally gratifying. One way to do this is to seek promotion or apply for a specialty assignment such as the

SWAT team, the field training program, the canine squad, and so on.

You are encouraging when your mate puts in for a promotion or specialty assignment. You may be hoping to see him or her off the street in a safer job or off shift work so that you can have a more normal schedule. You're probably hoping for additional money so you can start a family or buy a bigger house. However, specialty assignments may require undercover work, more hours away from home, or increased exposure to danger.

You and your cop probably believe that hard work and mastery will be rewarded. Both of you have sacrificed significant time together so that your officer could demonstrate his or her dedication to the job and to getting ahead. At first, neither of you really expects success; rather, you regard the process as a way to gain experience for the future. But each successive competition increases your expectations, and each failure is harder to take.

I can usually tell when a promotional process is happening. Officers are eager to work on new projects. Uniforms are spiffier than usual. Everyone is looking around, suspicious that each other's every move is a political strategy to curry favor with superiors. The competition is palpable, and this is uncomfortable because it pits people against each other, people who depend upon each other in significant ways. The whole process takes place in a fishbowl with lists and ratings posted for all to see.

Officers and their families are not well prepared for the anxiety and disappointment that accompany getting ahead. We teach officers street survival skills, but we fail to teach them how to survive in their own organizations. Police organizations are shaped like pyramids, with very little room at the top. There is approximately one supervisory position for every eight patrol officers, and only 5% will be promoted to an executive rank. Promotional opportunities are especially scarce in small departments, and departments of 50 or fewer officers make up nearly 90% of all police agencies.

In our culture, upward mobility, accumulation, prestige, and status are the ways in which we judge our success in life and measure our self-worth. Men, in particular, have been saddled with this judgment. Male officers may feel guilty if their wives have to work, especially after requiring the family to put up with all the other pressures that go along with having a cop as a husband or father. Female officers may feel sad and regretful for postponing marriage or childbearing. Both may be devastated by the sacrifices they made to get ahead. A promotional failure brings all these decisions into question.

Police psychologist Ira Grossman (1994) calls promotional disappointments "injuries without violence." Officers are expected to stifle their anger and shame and quietly accept the results. This is what happened to Lew. He was the personal favorite of all street cops—a wise, witty, and concerned man with 15 years of street experience. He had put in for promotion to sergeant every year for the last seven years. He wanted to give up, but he found it hard to resist the pressure from his fellow officers, who complained about how green all the recently promoted people were and how much they hated working for them.

The truth of the matter was that Lew had only a high school diploma and no experience beyond street patrol. His department had experienced a lot of turnover and was anticipating several retirements in the managerial ranks. They were desperately in need of college-educated officers who could be promoted to fill those managerial positions, or they would be forced to hire from outside, something they wanted to avoid.

Lew was tired of fighting the impossible odds, and so was his family. He finally declined to put in for promotion again because he knew it was futile. Though he was privately bitter about forsaking the opportunity to be a career sergeant, he ultimately felt calmer about accepting the reality of his situation.

Police administrators amplify this problem when they encourage officers to apply for career-enhancing positions despite the limited opportunities. When cops fail to be assigned to a specialty or fail to be promoted, they are encouraged to work harder and seek more education. Rarely are they honestly told about the reality of their future potential or given other ways to find reward and renewal in their work. To the contrary, when officers give up on the promotional process, they are often written off as apathetic deadbeats.

There is a lot that police agencies could do to improve this system but little that you as the family can affect, except to learn to cope sensibly with the ups and the downs.

PHASE THREE: DEALING WITH DISILLUSIONMENT

Just a few years ago, the veteran was an idealistic supercop out to solve crime and make this a better world. Now he or she believes that the best that can be done is to maintain order and hold the line. The judicial system doesn't work, criminals have the advantage over cops, and victims' needs don't count. Neither the community nor the department understands or appreciates the police. Politics, rather than fairness or justice, dominate the scene. The media are 10 times more interested in the occasional police scandal than the thousands of everyday acts of courage and persistence. To make matters worse, your cop has probably discovered a few gray hairs, your children might be approaching adolescence, and your parents are showing signs of old age.

An officer may be buffered against such negativity if he or she has been promoted or has received a valued specialty assignment. This is not to say that officers who are promoted are without problems. It is a shock to many cops who have automatically assumed they wanted to be on that uphill track that their hard-won promotion turned out to be a source of discomfort.

Take Davita, for example. When Davita was promoted to sergeant, she was ecstatic. It was, therefore, a shock and a surprise when she sensed her carpool buddies were acting coolly toward her, and their usually rowdy and raucous conversations had grown stilted. When she confronted her friends, they told her they could no longer trust her because she was now a supervisor. They worried that whatever they said to her, whether about themselves or someone else, could be used against them in future competitive processes or in their yearly evaluations. Davita was astonished; these were her friends and confidants. She hadn't changed at all.

To add insult to injury, at the time she made sergeant, Davita heard complaints that her promotion was based not on merit but, rather, on the fact that her department was under pressure to promote a minority member in order to satisfy community groups who monitored the status of women and minorities in city government. Davita felt she got absolutely no credit for her hard work or competency. This drove her closer to the other supervisors and cemented the rupture between her and her friends.

Abe had also worked hard to be promoted. He and his family had sacrificed a lot so that he could build his reputation as a tireless worker, willing to go the extra mile. They did without him when he was studying for promotional exams and when he was finishing his college degree. Once he was promoted, Abe realized he had known little about the reality of his new position. He had few supervisory duties and spent most of his time working on paper projects for the chief—budget preparation, reports for the board of supervisors, and the like. He felt stifled being in an office and longed for the street action. He didn't like being on the bottom of the managerial heap and felt he got blamed for things beyond his control. He had imagined that as a manager he would have more authority to make a difference. In fact, he had less.

Abe stewed about this for a year and talked about it with his family. They told him that they loved him for who he was, not his rank, and that his misery was of his own making. Abe then decided to ask for a voluntary demotion back to the rank of sergeant, where he was happiest and most productive. He raised a lot of eyebrows, but clearly he did the right thing for himself and his family.

There are many stresses attached to successful promotion: Police chiefs are among the most isolated and vilified employees in a police organization. I have known chiefs who have literally barricaded themselves in their offices because every time they ventured out they were bombarded with complaints about everything, ranging from patrol cars to staffing levels. I have known chiefs who were spied on, shot at, and slandered. The higher the rank, the bigger the target and the more nights out eating overcooked chicken at public events or trying to stay alert at mind-deadening city council meetings that last past midnight. Police chiefs appear to be all-powerful to their employees, but they often feel powerless in their dealings with city managers and city councils. The buck stops with the chief during a scandal or a community controversy; unfortunately, it also lands on his or her family as they struggle with the anguish of public scrutiny.

Despite these stresses, officers who have been promoted or placed in a long-term special assignment seem to fare better over the long haul than their unpromoted coworkers. Their self-esteem is stronger, they are politically more powerful, and they are socially more skillful. They are also more committed to the job, are more burdened with responsibility, and work longer hours, all of which may put additional strain on their family life.

These years may generate an identity crisis for cops who don't get promoted, placing them at risk for becoming frustrated, bitter, and cynical. Their self-image is tarnished, and they may doubt their own capabilities as they watch people pass them by on the promotional ladder. It takes an extremely confident person to gracefully be supervised by someone he or she once trained as a rookie.

Many cops settled into their career early in life, married young, and accumulated a middle-aged mountain of financial responsibilities by the time they hit their early 30s. Now they feel locked into policing but locked out of the rewards that policing once offered. The career that promised them 20 to 25 years of fulfillment seems over in 10. The compensation that was once such a draw is now a trap—what other work will pay as well? How can they risk financial security by changing careers?

During this period, all past decisions may come into question. Why did he or she choose this career, marry young, fail to finish college, work so hard for a master's degree, have kids, not have kids? How competent is he or she really? Where did all the money go? Where did all the time go? Is he or she a good parent, a good spouse, a good cop?

This is suffering. Officers may doubt that anyone understands or cares about their welfare and what they have to deal with on the street. They become fixated on personal concerns, especially salary, schedules, and other compensation issues. Wages equal self-worth. Appreciation of their work is so hard to come by that some cops will begin to file for 15 minutes of overtime in a job that years ago they might have performed for free.

Those who are deeply disillusioned may become increasingly irritated and critical of the organization they once naively regarded as a benevolent parent. They see their jobs as the most important, yet least acknowledged. They have only criticism for supervisors and administrators who do nothing right and never know what is going on. One wonders how they would have felt being promoted to this despised group of "incompetents." Their world has been reduced to "us" and "them," and *they* are worthy only of contempt. People are "perps" and "slime bags." Successful cops are "brown nosers" and "fast trackers." Racism, sexism, and all the other "isms" that support an egocentric worldview are rampant. Victims, except for children and old people, are seen as fools who deserved what they got.

During this phase, frustrated cops may contemplate changing jobs only to be confronted by their lack of education, their abundant financial needs, and the nagging fear that being a cop has damaged their capacity to comfortably socialize with civilians. Over and over again I hear cops say, "I can't do anything but police work," which greatly underestimates the skills they have accumulated but cannot translate into language that is understood by the civilian world. With no programs in place to assist in the transition out of policing, many disgruntled officers settle in to wait out the years before retirement in apathy and depression.

Your family may become a target for displacing the helplessness and frustration your cop feels at work. Your own profession may be placing big demands on your time and energy, leaving little time for either of you to focus on your marriage. The situation might appear hopeless; it may seem easier to separate or divorce than to resolve such serious problems. For some people, divorce will be the right answer because there is not enough trust or goodwill left to offset the stresses. But for most, it is important to hang in and remember this, too, is a phase that will pass.

Mick hung in through the bad times. At age 47, he was still pushing a patrol car. He wore glasses that he was afraid of losing in a fight, and while his back wasn't bad enough for a medical retirement, it hurt him all the time. He was bitter because he had never received the recognition he felt he deserved, and he would sit in the back of briefings, taking verbal pot shots at everyone and everything. His cynicism infected others on his shift, and he was generally regarded as a problem employee. The young, "hot dog" cops referred to him as a "slug" and a "blowhard."

Mick's wife, Katherine, was caught up in her own pursuits and worn out from listening to his complaints. The only thing they had in common was their children, who were almost grown. They had started avoiding each other because each felt helpless to resolve their problems. It had been years since they had taken a vacation without the kids. They justified this by saying they didn't have the money, but in truth, they were afraid of the silences between them whenever they were alone.

When their teenage son got into some trouble with the law, the probation officer required the entire family to seek family counseling. They stayed in counseling for a long, hard year, but counseling broke the ice. Katherine learned that while she was not responsible for solving Mick's problems, she was responsible for not getting dragged down or disillusioned by his negativity. One of the things she most hated about their life was how many civilian friends had dropped away, perhaps because of Mick's cynicism. She began looking for ways to make new friends for herself.

Mick began to deal with his depression and frustration. He had been regarding retirement as a magic pill that would solve years of accumulated problems. He discovered that his family needed his attention now and might not be around when he retired.

As his depression lifted, Mick got less irritable at home and at work. He began to participate in recreational activities and take up exercise. He and Katherine took a long-overdue trip together. He had a little more energy because he was less depressed, and he found other ways to feel successful and satisfied. He got philosophical about work and decided that being a mediocre cop was good enough for him. It was important for him to plan for the future and concentrate on getting to retirement safely.

PHASE FOUR: COMING TO A CROSSROAD

Lynda and Miguel were at a crossroad: They had to find a way to renew their interests in work and each other or sink into indifference and apathy. They rarely went out, and when they did, they only went to other cops' houses, where all they did was talk about administrators and "perps" as though they were one and the same. Lynda tried to pick up Miguel's spirits: She urged him to take up golf. Nothing worked.

After months of thinking about this, Lynda told Miguel that she understood that he was having a rough time at work, that it was clear he didn't know what to do to make it better for himself, and that neither did she. As a matter of fact, trying to help him made her realize that she, too, was feeling lost and bored. She told him that she had decided to enroll in a painting class, something she had wanted to do for a long time.

Miguel objected. He told her it was dangerous on campus at night; he protested that they didn't have the money for art supplies; he wondered why his company wasn't enough for her; he asked who would cook his dinner. Lynda listened patiently and told Miguel that it was not her intention to abandon him, but if she didn't find something that gave shape and meaning to her life, she would become depressed.

On her first night of class, Miguel had some "emergency" overtime and couldn't get the car home on time. Lynda felt so discouraged she almost gave up. But she had anticipated some countermoves on Miguel's part, so she asked her neighbor for a lift and begged a ride home from a fellow student. She would have taken a taxi if she had to.

She repeatedly told Miguel that she was sorry he felt angry and hurt but that she needed to do this for herself and hoped he would understand. She didn't tell him how to fill his time or lecture him about getting a hobby.

Miguel was mad. He thought about having an affair; he began to go out with his friends and come home drunk. Nothing seemed to knock Lynda off course. Miguel felt like a three-year-old who was pitching a long tantrum. He was mad at himself for being so dependent on Lynda that he couldn't let her have a night to herself. He realized that he was in a terrible rut and was jealous that Lynda had something of her own that made her happy. He began to look around for something that would add to his life. He visited a retired cop friend who was a woodworker, and he started learning woodcraft. Soon, he set up a small workshop in his garage. Lynda bought him some tools and a subscription to a woodworking magazine for his birthday, and by Christmas he had made simple gifts for all their friends and an easel for Lynda.

Woodworking presented Miguel with a new set of problems, problems over which he had some control. It gave him the opportunity to complete a task and wind up with a tangible product, something police work rarely provides. He preferred these new "problems" to his old ones, and consequently, the old ones lost some of their charge.

Most couples have to work at renewing their longtime relationship and finding things in common to fill their time. When love was new, she may have been willing to sit through a baseball game, and he may have been willing to go to the ballet to please her. But as time passes, our needs and tastes are more finely shaped, and the pressure of too little time requires us to choose carefully how we spend that time. We are less willing to do what we don't want to do. This is not a police-only problem. Houses and relationships are always in need of renewing and repairing.

Officers who are at crossroads in their careers have probably come to accept the reality of their situation and the futility of tilting at windmills. They see the cost of perpetually assaulting or resisting something that will barely change. They accept that it is time to invoke the Serenity prayer from Alcoholics Anonymous: "God grant me the serenity to accept those things I cannot change, the courage to change those things I cannot accept, and the wisdom to know the difference."

Rather than looking at past disappointments, your cop is now probably focusing on the benefits of retiring at about age 50. Fifty doesn't seem so old anymore or so far in the future. Cops at the crossroad begin to make plans, to consider what to do next. They have a more realistic view of the job and of their own limitations. They are more philosophical; they know someone else will get the bad guy if they don't. They are less inclined to take risks.

At this crossroad, cops usually accept the fact they are no longer promotable and look for other ways to satisfy personal goals and stay interested in work. They realize that the grass is not necessarily greener on the other side; that most agencies, not just their own, have limited opportunities for promotion and few alternative methods of seeking self-renewal, personal development, and new learning. They stop looking elsewhere and look inward to satisfy these universal needs for stimulation and emotional gratification. They may set new goals that are unrelated to work by taking up hobbies or developing a renewed interest in their families or in their religion.

This can be a time when senior officers enjoy the perks of their experience. They have little left to lose. Unless they commit some crime or an atrocious act of negligence, they are unlikely to be fired or laid off. They are out of the political rat race, which gives them freedom to be themselves and not worry as much about the impact of everything they do or say. They should be thinking about the legacy they want to leave behind when they retire and how they will accomplish this in their remaining years on the force. It may not be the heroic legacy they dreamed of as a rookie but a realistic legacy seasoned with their years of experience.

They can take an interest in younger officers or develop an expertise that does not require a promotion to implement such as range master, crime scene I.D., accident investigation, and so on. They can apply for specialty training. They can involve themselves in "kiddie cop" details. Often looked at as second-class policing, mature officers recognize the potential of working with young people. They can take up a cause, such as the development of a peer support network or a trauma intervention team. They can start projects for the union, such as developing and institutionalizing ways to reward senior officers or support people moving toward retirement. They can start projects to stay in touch with disabled cops who are isolated at home.

Todd provides a good example of using initiative to bring meaning into the remaining years of a long career. He spent many of his last years assembling and updating a computerized list of all the previous retirees and their dates of service. This gave the department a sense of its own history, acknowledged the people who had gone before, and reconnected them to each other and to the department since the department now had an accurate mailing list for inviting these retired officers to events honoring newly retired people. It also gave Todd a good excuse to learn more about computers, a useful skill and hobby for his retirement.

Another officer, Burt, wrote and distributed a research report about retirement, summarizing both the psychological and financial considerations he felt were important. It was so useful, he was asked to run some seminars for other departments and to share it with human resources personnel.

The advent of community policing presents another avenue for the senior officer. It gives him or her increased opportunity and authority to develop projects in concert with community residents. Community policing, when properly implemented and not just a series of slogans, encourages and rewards officers for their initiative in discovering and remedying community concerns. In other words, your officer may have the opportunity to come full circle and rev up the idealism that fueled his or her early days on the job. He or she can once again become a protector of the community, working closely with community groups who are eager for help and respectful of the years of expertise your cop has accumulated. Working together is a powerful way to break down stereotypes—to reduce the cynicism your cop may have toward others and modify the distorted view so many citizens have of cops.

Tips for Career Management

- Monitor your stress levels and develop positive coping skills while you're young. Older workers in high-stress jobs are vulnerable to health problems when they rely on risky coping behaviors like drinking and gambling to manage stress.
- Determine early on what success and gratification mean to you and your mate. How do money, prestige, and status affect your definition of success?
- Look for rewards and satisfactions that aren't based on upward mobility and accumulation. Such rewards are more often found in family life and personal pursuits than at work. People on their death beds rarely regret not having gone to their offices more often.
- Talk with your spouse about your mutual goals in life while you still have time to make long-range plans that don't rely on promotion or increased income. Sit down together and write up a family plan: Set realistic, achievable, and manageable goals for five-year increments from now through retirement.
- Plan your finances from the beginning so that your cop can leave his or her job if it becomes unbearable. Avoid becoming financially handcuffed to the police salary or a far-off pension.

(cont.)

(continued from previous page)

Save money from *year one*. Avoid living beyond your means or confusing material accumulation with genuine satisfaction. Create a backup plan that answers this question: What will we do if this cop job doesn't work out in 5, 10, or 15 years?

- Don't blame yourself or each other for disappointment. There are always more candidates than open slots. Don't assume—or let your cop assume—that because he or she failed a competitive process he or she is a failure.

- Develop social networks in fields besides law enforcement, in case you need them.

- Continue with your education and encourage your spouse to get a broad-based education that qualifies him or her for other fields.

- Plan, plan, plan. If you have not begun planning for retirement, start now. Begin investigating the realities of your financial situation and projecting your future economic needs against your future income.

- If you or your mate is nearing retirement, decide now what you want to do and how you will spend your time. Will you both be working, or will one of you be at home? If so, what issues does this raise? What are your expectations of each other? It is beyond the scope of this book to go into the specifics of planning for retirement, but there are excellent books to consult (see Recommended Reading in the Resources section).

- Encourage your officer to begin considering his or her legacy about five years before his or her retirement date. It is best to retire on a positive note, feeling we have made a difference in the lives of people we have met. Look for positive examples of how others have done this.

CHAPTER 4

ORGANIZATIONAL STRESS

Looking for Love
in All the Wrong Places

> The truth shall set you free, but first
> it will piss you off.
> —ANONYMOUS

When I walk into a police agency, I often feel as if I have brought my briefcase to a battlefield. I say to myself that what I really need now is a flak jacket instead of a flip chart. It is like war inside some agencies. Administrators treat their employees like demanding, willful, impulsive adolescents who cannot be trusted, and the employees regard their administrators as unpredictable, withholding, and punitive parents who cannot be depended upon for support. What is missing in all this mudslinging is any recognition that all ranks must meet challenging and complex responsibilities, and all cops have strengths and weaknesses.

Strife can erupt anywhere in a police organization, and it usually does. Labor and management are at odds over working conditions and benefits. Male officers are angry at female officers and vice versa. The black officers' association and the white officers' association are fighting. The detective bureau is unhappy with how patrol officers write reports, and patrol officers think the detectives hoard information. One cop thinks he works harder, answers more calls, and does more paperwork than anyone else on his squad, while his squadmates complain he can't be found when needed. The sergeants can't stand the lieutenants, and the lieutenants think the sergeants are flakes. The captain is angry because the chief is micromanaging and has kicked back his council report for the fourth revision. The cops are angry with the way communicators dispatch calls for service at the same time that the communicators are furious with the cops for not answering. Two communicators can't stand working the same shift together. The front desk people are angry with the data-entry folks. Clerks are frustrated because the cops don't check the right boxes on their reports. The detectives are angry because the D.A. won't file on a perfectly good case. The D.A. is angry because the case report is sloppy and weak. Some citizens are angry because the cops won't put up a stop sign on their corner. The city manager is angry at the police union because negotiations are creating bad publicity. The chief is angry at being misquoted by the media, and everyone is angry with the chief.

Someone, somewhere in every police department I have ever visited is upset about something. Perhaps he got what he considers to be a bogus, trumped-up citizen's complaint. Maybe she is the object of an internal affairs investigation or the recipient of a performance improvement plan. Or he might be assigned to light duty when he wants to work or to work when he thinks he needs light duty. Probably she didn't get the commendation she thought she deserved or had to watch while some undeserving, but politically correct, kiss-up did.

To understand what makes cops tick, you have to know as much about where they work as what they do. Cops work in bureaucracies, and these bureaucracies create stress that far exceeds the stress they experience in the line of duty. Danger is not an everyday occurrence for most cops, but organizational stress and office politics are. Cops are taught how to deal with danger as though it happens every day, but rarely, if ever, are they taught to anticipate—and, in turn to manage—the daily grind of a bureaucratic system. I have, half jokingly, suggested that my colleagues who screen police applicants would provide a much needed service if they were to also screen agencies so they could guide prospective applicants toward the agencies that were the most respectful and supportive of their employees.

WHAT CAUSES ORGANIZATIONAL STRESS?

Almost all people who work in organizations complain of organizational stress. Over the years my colleagues and I have identified several primary causes of organizational stress in law enforcement.

- Inadequate training
- Poor supervision
- Poor equipment
- Unfair workload distribution
- Inadequate rewards, compensation, or acknowledgment
- Poor communication
- Lack of administrative support
- Politics
- Unfair shift assignments
- Few family-friendly policies
- Unfair disciplinary practices
- Poorly managed change
- Favoritism
- Poor leadership
- Lack of clarity and feedback about roles, expectations, and responsibilities

What does organizational stress mean to you and your family? It will be a source of continuous strain for you and your mate, the topic of many dinner-table conversations, and the subject of much pillow talk. Research has shown that spouses are vicariously affected by organizational stress, discouraged by the impact office politics has on their spouses' careers, resentful of the degree to which the organization intrudes into their family life, and angry that the organization seems to care so little about what families need in order to thrive.

Organizational stress takes a toll on the health and well-being of all employees—line level, middle management, and administration. I have spent most of my career thinking, consulting, and writing about organizational stress in law enforcement, starting with my doctoral dissertation. I have concluded that organizations cannot permanently fix the causes of organizational stress, but they can learn to manage them better.

ORGANIZATIONAL DILEMMAS

It is hard for police officers to properly serve the public when they believe themselves to be poorly supported by their agencies. On the other hand, the definition of what it means to be supportive varies greatly, depending on whether you are talking to a manager, a supervisor, a line-level officer, a civilian employee, the mayor, a member of the police review board, or a citizen.

There is continuous debate over how to fairly balance individual and organizational responsibility for the health and well-being of police officers. For example, should a police department pay cops to stop smoking or lose weight, or is that the individual's responsibility? Should departments provide female officers with paid maternity leave, or is the decision to have children a responsibility to be borne by the officer herself?

One of the most unique aspects of a police organization is that the lowest-ranked workers, the line-level troops, are the most visible, powerful, and autonomous. But, rarely do they feel as powerful as they are. In fact, much of the time, they experience the terrible dilemma of being simultaneously powerful and powerless: powerful because their every action has potentially critical consequences; powerless because they are constantly scrutinized, supervised, and reined in by their own department and by the community in ways that can be irritating, humiliating, and sometimes irrelevant to their actual job performance. For example, cops are often besieged with legalistic, paternalistic directives regarding the length of their hair, the neatness of their mailboxes, or how shiny their badges are. Their reports are summarily rejected for minor spelling errors, and too rarely do they get acknowledged for the arrest or the investigation that generated the report. Professional police officers ought to be able to turn in neat, correctly spelled, and complete reports; but it is understandably aggravating to make a good arrest, get a crook off the street, and have your sergeant pay more attention to the fact that you forgot to check all the boxes on the face sheet. There is no question in my mind that cops must be held accountable for their actions and their time, but to hold them accountable without simultaneously providing them with support is not right and doesn't work. It only creates resentment and rebelliousness.

How best to provide that support is often not obvious. John's experience is a case in point. John was in a hot foot pursuit with his gun drawn when it accidentally discharged into the ground. After he arrested the fleeing suspect, he went back and recovered the bullet. No one was hurt and no citizens called to complain.

John was immediately recalled to the department, put in seclusion, and given a blood test to determine if he had been drinking or using drugs. This is standard procedure in his department, one that is designed to protect John and his department from accusations of a cover-up if someone were later to report being injured and file a lawsuit—as sometimes happens when a bullet is accidentally fired and not recovered or ricochets into a nearby building. Everyone agreed that the need to take a sample of John's blood was procedural only; no one had any reason to suspect that John was under the influence of anything other than his desire to catch the crook.

John was hurt and angry. He felt like a criminal and a victim at the same time. As a matter of fact, he felt the criminal had more rights than he did. This same crook had gotten into a fight with an officer from a neighboring district a year ago and had bitten the officer on the arm, breaking his skin. Because the suspect was an intravenous drug user, there was reason to think he might be HIV-infected, but no one could force him to give blood. The injured officer and his family were very worried that the officer might have contracted AIDS. This affected the couple's sex life and the family's emotional life. The officer elected to begin azathioprene AZT (azidothymidine, now known as zidovudine) therapy immediately and suffer the side effects of the medication rather than wait six months for his second AIDS test, which fortunately, turned out to be negative. All of this might have been avoided had the suspect voluntarily agreed to be tested.

Back to John. Should John have been ordered to take a blood test because there was a chance that someone would later claim injury or question his actions? Should the department open itself to possible accusations of a cover-up by not requiring the test? Whose needs take priority? Can everyone's concerns be fairly addressed at the same time? Would John have been more receptive if the process had been handled differently, or was he so hypervigilant after the accidental discharge that he misunderstood and catastrophized his department's every action?

These questions can only be answered on a case-by-case basis and probably never to the satisfaction of all involved. What is important for families to know and understand is that organizational stress will affect a cop and will hurt and agitate him or her more deeply than the crooks on the street. Cops who go through something like this may not be able to sleep. They may talk about feeling like criminals or victims—helpless and out of control. They may go in search of villains, people to blame. They may seek revenge or simply shut down and refuse to do any work. They may act out. They will probably be inconsolable for a time.

Cops expect crooks to try to hurt them. But when they feel as if their own organizations are turning on them, it is like being stabbed in the back by a member of the family. Cops expect their agencies to stand by them and support them against hostile outsiders. They want to believe that their agency will function as a surrogate family with just, caring parents and supportive siblings who fairly share the rewards and misfortunes of life. This expectation is so powerful it often obscures the fact that police administrators serve many masters and must take the rights and needs of all into account. It is ironic that the same organization that can be accused of abandoning cops can also be accused by the community of overprotecting and covering up for them.

ONE SIN IS WORTH A THOUSAND GOOD DEEDS: DISCIPLINARY ACTION

One of the most stressful events that can occur in an officer's life is receiving disciplinary action. Hypervigilance amplifies and prolongs this stress, making it worse than it already is.

Hypervigilant cops have compromised their ability to tell genuinely lethal situations from those that are not lethal. They are constantly looking for conspiracies and plots against the troops behind every management move. Not all management directives are wise, thoughtful, or effective, but they are also not *always* misdirected or mean-spirited.

Benny's case illustrates how painful disciplinary action is for the officer and his or her family and how hypervigilance magnifies the pain. Benny was a gung-ho street cop who was involved in a vehicle pursuit and subsequent foot chase of a carjacker. It took 15 minutes for Benny and his partner, Ray, to capture this man, who had Herculean strength. Ray and Benny were exhausted. They had run through so many backyards and jumped so many fences that they lost track of where they were and couldn't give dispatch an accurate address for backup. They knew they were on their own until other officers could locate them or someone nearby heard the noise and called 911.

They wrestled the suspect to the ground, and Ray had one handcuff on him but couldn't get hold of his other hand, which was hidden from sight. What happened next was unclear. The man claimed Benny purposefully and repeatedly kicked him in the stomach and the face. Benny didn't deny it but said he did so because he thought the man had a knife in his hidden hand, although no weapon was ever found. Ray sided with the suspect, saying he thought he had the situation under control, and Benny had overreacted. The situation had ugly racial overtones, since Benny is white and Ray and the suspect are African American.

The consequences of this event hit everyone. The chief and the city manager were besieged with angry citizens, consumer action groups, and the media, all of whom had their own agendas. The suspect's family retained a lawyer and demanded a hearing.

The other officers were devastated. Benny and Ray were both popular, and their fellow cops felt forced to choose sides. One of Benny's good friends, Frank, was put in charge of the internal affairs investigation. Several of his friends were required to give testimony about that evening's actions. They understood the need to be interviewed but were uncomfortable when Frank began asking them about past incidents involving Benny. They felt protective toward Benny and were disturbed to give "aid to the enemy," which is how they regarded the internal affairs investigators. They talked among themselves about how investigative strategies ordinarily used with suspects were now being used against them. They worried about being set up for disciplinary action. They fumed that things they had said off the record to Frank had become part of the investigation. They also feared reprisals for saying anything bad against Ray because they thought he was on the fast track for promotion and would eventually wind up supervising them.

Frank was regarded as a turncoat even though he was doing his assigned job. He was greeted with silence in the hallways, and people stopped inviting him along on coffee breaks. He had trouble sleeping, and his stomach ached constantly.

Benny felt he had no rights. He could be charged criminally or civilly, and he was subject to administrative action as well. He was absolutely convinced that his career was over, and he was racked with guilt for failing his family.

At home alone during the investigation, Benny spent his days depressed and crying. When his wife, Carole, came back from work, he would try to perk up for her sake, but he never could hide the depths of his despair. All day long he catastrophized that this was truly the end of his career and that he would be fired. He worried constantly about how he could support his family. He couldn't imagine what he would do if he weren't a cop, and he couldn't picture drawing an equivalent salary since he had only a high school education. He felt guilty because he thought Carole was being punished for his alleged misdeeds.

He was given to ruminating and obsessively second-guessing his judgment on that night. He wondered how he could function as a cop in today's world, where suspects had all the rights and fellow cops couldn't be trusted to stand up for one another.

The investigation took six months to complete. When it was finally over, Benny was demoted and given three months off without pay, which equaled a fine of several thousand dollars. The cost of his demotion far exceeded the fine as he calculated how much less he would earn over the remaining years of his career and how this lower pay status would negatively affect the formula used to calculate his retirement pension.

When Benny finally returned to work, nine months after the incident, he was nearly paralyzed with anxiety. The chief called him into his office and asked what he could do to help. He offered to give Benny time off to get counseling and told him that if he could change his attitude and deal better with stress, Benny could expect his support. He was serious about these changes and put Benny on a performance plan that stated any further sustained complaints could be grounds for immediate termination.

When Benny sought counseling, he did so on his own even though the chief had offered to pay for it with department funds. He told me he didn't believe a word of what his chief had said. He thought Ray had lied, and he didn't know whom to trust anymore. None of his administrators understood anything about the street, and because of this, they failed to appreciate how dangerous things were. Benny was afraid that he had become so cautious about taking any action at all that he was compromising his officer safety standards.

According to Benny, minority groups made all white males so uncomfortable they couldn't function. He had lost his self-confidence, as well as the joy and spontaneity he used to feel at work. He thought everyone was watching him. He was afraid to do anything but drive around because if he had to take any action at all, he was scared he would do the wrong thing. He was sure everyone, the chief especially, was waiting for him to mess up. He couldn't sleep, and he cried uncontrollably in my office. Carole got pregnant and had a miscarriage.

One day, Benny received a citizen's complaint. He was frantic. This was it; this was all the department needed to fire him. His wife was on sick leave and couldn't work. They would be destitute, and he would be unable to support her. He declared he would get a divorce in order to give Carole another chance with a man who could be a better husband than he was. I asked him how he knew his career was over. What evidence was there that people were waiting to fire him? He had no evidence at all, except the evidence of his own emotions: If he was afraid, there must be something to fear; if he was suspicious, people must be plotting against him; and so on. We worked together on thought-stopping techniques to break his negative thought patterns. We rehearsed how he could deal assertively with this new complaint and not mix it up with the last one because they were different. I helped him to stop jacking himself up with a steady patter of anxiety-provoking "what ifs."

As it turned out, this new complaint was unfounded. It was a simple matter and quickly settled. Benny had to admit that he was treated fairly and got to see how he had exaggerated and inflated his difficulties. Benny told his chief how anxious he had been, and his chief got a chance to tell Benny again that he had no interest in torturing or firing him. He encouraged Benny to put in for positions that would get him out of the field because he had been on the street for nearly 15 years. Benny was astonished. He thought his chances for special assignment or promotion were absolutely nil.

I may never know what actually happened in Benny's incident. Like so many police actions, it happened in the dark, there were split-second decisions to be made, and everyone, including the suspect, was exhausted and scared. Was Benny deliberately brutal? I doubt it. Was his department right to investigate the situation? Absolutely. Were they gunning for him? I don't think so. Would it have been better had the investigation gone faster? Certainly. Was Benny's discipline too harsh or too lenient? That depends on whom you ask.

Benny's story illustrates what is both painful and inevitable for cops. It is impossible to perform work with such serious consequences and avoid doing something that someone thinks is wrong. It is impossible to work as a cop and avoid making an honest mistake. It is impossible to work as a cop and avoid getting disciplined. Cops cannot and should not walk away when they are needed. But every time they take an action, they take a risk.

When your loved one receives discipline, be prepared. You can predict it will feel undeserved and like a betrayal. It is a normal human reflex to be defensive when attacked, and a disciplinary action almost always feels like an attack. Part of a good defense is a strong offense, and under the circumstances, your cop will likely be inclined to reduce an excruciatingly complex organizational dilemma to a simple black-or-white, "with me or against me" principle. I have never known a cop who welcomed any internal investigation as a way of getting to the bottom of a problem and learning whether there was something he or she did wrong and could do better next time. It simply doesn't happen that way.

As part of your cop's support system, you can be helpful by being a good, empathetic listener. You don't have to try the case in your house, dispute or agree with the facts, give advice, call up the chief, telephone the newspapers, explain the department to your mate or your mate to the department, or do anything other than be a good listener, which is hard enough work. This is especially so under the circumstances because taking action is an effective way to relieve stress. Unfortunately, many actions decided under stress are wrong and create more problems than they solve.

You will also need to control your own anxiety about possible termination or suspension and the subsequent loss of pay. Under this kind of stress, your mate will probably not be as much of a support system for you as you are for him or her. Find someone, perhaps another police spouse, you can talk to, someone who will help you contain your anxiety, stop you from catastrophizing, and let you express those emotions you may be holding back at home. This person can help you develop a game plan for coping with a lengthy investigation or disciplinary action.

Not every disciplinary action involves possible criminal charges or is necessarily preceded by an internal affairs investigation, but most serious allegations of a violation of department regulations do require some form of investigation and a written report, both of which can take an unbelievably long time to prepare. And any investigation becomes massively stressful if the media are involved.

THE SECOND INJURY: BUREAUCRATIC FRIENDLY FIRE

Benny's agency had no other choice but to investigate his incident. I know Benny felt his chief was out to get him, but I couldn't see what his chief had to gain from subjecting any of his officers to a grueling and dispiriting process. And, after the process was through, his chief seemed to make a genuine effort to get Benny back on his feet and retain him as a cop.

Unfortunately, I have known officers who were mistreated after a job-related incident and virtually hounded out of their departments. This is the nonviolent equivalent of friendly fire. The people you expect to support you, who may have promised to support you, seem to turn on you when you need them most. Psychologists call this "the second injury." What is so devastating about second injuries is that they are largely preventable.

My first encounter with a second injury was with Kent. Kent was an experienced cop with a reputation as an independent thinker. He had been shot in the line of duty after surprising some survivalists who were poaching deer in the rural district he patrolled. The poachers opened fire, hitting him twice and disabling his shooting hand. Kent lay defenseless for several minutes, waiting for his backup unit and an ambulance to arrive.

When the police chief arrived at the hospital, the first thing he did was blame Kent for his injuries. He thought Kent should have waited for a backup unit when he discovered the poachers' truck, but Kent knew his backup unit was 10 minutes away and feared the poachers would leave as soon as they saw him. The chief, who was an acting chief, apparently wanted to avoid media questions about staffing levels in his department, which was a hot political issue.

Kent's wife, Elise, was at his bedside. She couldn't believe the chief was more concerned about looking good for the media than he was about Kent's injuries. Kent was everything to her, but to the chief he was merely "a jerk with bullet holes in him who was going to take the rap for everything!"

Thus began a prolonged battle between Kent and his department—a battle over responsibility, blame, lack of acknowledgment, and compensation. Kent felt totally abandoned by his administration as they fought him at every turn. The initial outpouring of support from his coworkers soon faded as they grew tired of the fight and impatient with Kent's long recovery. It was as though looking at his injuries and his grievances was a mirror of what might happen to them some day. It was too painful to contemplate. Kent felt dropped like a hot potato. He counted this as another unexpected and devastating injury.

The battle between Kent and his department gravely impaired his physical and mental recovery and all but destroyed his motivation to get back to work. In the end, he wore out his wife, lost all his money, destroyed his mental health, and was beaten down by the worker's compensation bureaucracy, which has become the injurious adversarial system it was designed to avoid. It took 10 years to get his life back together. When I met him he was just getting back on his feet and trying to start a new business. He was wiser—but no less bitter: "The people who shot me shot me because I was a cop, not because I was Kent. The police department shot Kent."

It is hard to know if a little respect and human kindness delivered at his hospital bedside would have spared Kent and his department years of emotional and financial drain. Words have enormous power to wound. There are not enough pages in this book to recount all the stories I have heard about the damage done by careless remarks made during moments of high stress and anxiety. The price of such carelessness in a culture as unforgiving and vigilant as law enforcement is high. It degrades morale, creates emotional havoc, and courts financial ruin as emotionally wounded officers turn to lawsuits and disability retirements as a way to even the score and regain control and self-esteem.

The law enforcement culture is so rigid and unforgiving that bad situations are made worse for want of an apology. Minor disagreements can push the entire system into legalistic overdrive—people are prepared to do battle at the drop of a hat. Is this the natural consequence of hypervigilance? Or is it a reflection of how embattled and beleaguered many cops feel? They are at war with criminals, at war with drugs, at war with the community, at war with the media, at war with the courts, and when trouble comes, they are at war with each other.

Andy's situation illustrates this kind of knee-jerk reaction. Andy was a friendly, eager-to-please cop: a follower, not a leader. He took a blow to the head during a defensive tactics class and lost consciousness for several minutes. He came to in the ambulance, laughed the incident off with his usual self-deprecating jokes, went through a neurological examination in the emergency room, and was pronounced fit and ready to return to work after a few days' rest.

Two years later he was called to the scene of a traffic accident that was escalating into a riot and almost got sprayed with pepper gas by a fellow cop. At a debriefing later on, he broke down in tears; he was both frightened and angry.

Andy told his department psychologist that this relatively minor event brought back disturbing memories of a close call he had

had when he was a young reserve officer. He hadn't thought of the old incident in many years, and now, to his amazement, he was unable to stop thinking about it. The psychologist diagnosed him with a delayed posttraumatic stress response and recommended that Andy take a few days off from work, during which time they had several sessions and successfully reduced the severity of his symptoms. He was reassigned back to headquarters on modified duty, helping a commander prepare a report for the city council.

Within weeks, the psychologist received a frantic phone call from Andy, who was threatening to shoot his commander. Andy was angry and agitated. He claimed the commander was hounding him about finishing the report. Andy was again put on administrative leave and ordered to continue treatment. In therapy, he alternated between remorse and embarrassment for his threatening behavior and anger at the commander for being verbally abusive and disrespectful.

The psychologist took an extensive medical and social history. When he learned about Andy's head injury and loss of consciousness, he referred Andy to a neuropsychologist, who verified that Andy had sustained moderate brain damage when he was injured, impairing his ability to understand and retain new information—the very abilities he needed to complete his report. It also showed that Andy suffered from significant depression and a growing inability to control his emotions, all of which was substantiated by his wife.

Andy's psychologist believed that Andy's outbursts and threats were symptoms of his head injury. He was doubtful that Andy could return to work, but it was really too early to tell. He thought it important that Andy and his commander talk together.

These recommendations fell on deaf ears. Some of Andy's administrators didn't seem to value him as an employee. They implied that his 10 years of service were mediocre, and they appeared resentful at having to pay for his sick leave and rehabilitation services. They were doubtful of his injuries because of the delay in appearing, and they seemed suspicious of the psychologist's motives. Some admired the commander for his work ethic and strict supervision. They gave the psychologist the impression that they wished there were more employees like him and fewer like Andy.

Instead of trying to work out a mutually agreeable solution to this difficult situation or support a program that would address Andy's medical predicament, the department considered filing criminal charges against Andy for threatening a public official. They eventually granted Andy a medical retirement but not before they mounted a full internal affairs investigation that kept him, his family, and several other officers on edge for months.

I have to wonder what would have happened had Andy's department supported him. Would he have recovered from his disabilities sufficiently to pass a fitness-for-duty evaluation and return to work, which was what he wanted? Would the effort to retain him or retire him without a fight have been as costly, emotionally and financially, as the unsuccessful efforts to fire him?

Tips for Dealing with Organizational Stress

- Be proud of being a police family, but don't overidentify with the police role. Who you are as a family is determined by a lot more than the fact that a family member works in law enforcement. The more eggs you put into the police basket, the more dependent you are on the job for your quality of life and the more vulnerable you and your family are to changes, conflicts, or disappointments.
- Be prepared. Recognize that complaints and conflicts come with the territory.
- Pick your battles carefully. In a conflict between an individual and an organization, the individual is usually at a great disadvantage. Save your energy and your anger for the "big ones," if and when they occur.
- In the event of a complaint, investigation, or dispute with superiors, avoid getting hypervigilant along with your cop. Keep yourself from panicking.
- Join a support group or buddy up with a friend who can be there to support you while you support your cop.
- Know your legal rights and ask for help when you and your cop need it, but understand that legal victories are costly and

(cont.)

(continued from previous page)

sometimes hollow. Find lawyers who do not have an ax to grind and are open to mediation or negotiated settlements.

- Expect strong emotions. If you don't know how to respond, ask your mate what he or she needs or expects from you.
- Don't be a willing target. If your cop is displacing frustration or anger at the organization onto you or your family, be clear that this is unacceptable. Steer your partner back to the real problem. It may be easier to be mad at you than at an impersonal institution, but that is no excuse. If he or she can't use you as a sounding board, a compassionate witness, or a fellow problem solver, it is time to end the conversation.
- If you have questions about the part your cop may be playing in his or her problems, wait until the dust settles and emotions cool down to talk about it. Ask if the timing is okay to pose some hard questions that are bothering you, and then do so gently.
- If your cop is threatening physical violence toward the person he or she blames for all this stress, stay calm and say clearly that you think there are other, better options. Offer to talk the situation through. Try to get your cop to think through different scenarios: Ask how he would feel actually harming the person he is so angry at. If she says she'd feel great about getting even, ask if there would be negative consequences along with the positive? Ask if the pleasure is worth the price? Try to engage her in problem-solving discussions. Try to get him to talk about the hurt that often lies under anger. Buy yourself and your partner some time. People rarely make good decisions while they are in a rage. Take some time out: Go for a walk, take in a movie, and then talk about it. Avoid alcohol, which lowers inhibitions. Use your resources: Call friends, peer support personnel, the department psychologist, a police chaplain, your minister, or your local emergency mental health department.
- If that fails and your mate is getting ready to do something violent to another person, yourself included, call 911.

PART **II**

REMARKABLE
EVENTS

TRAUMA

CHAPTER 5

CRITICAL INCIDENTS, STRESS, AND TRAUMA

Work is, by its very nature, about violence—to
the spirit as well as to the body.
—STUDS TERKEL, *Working*

This is the story of two good friends, a police officer and a dispatcher. They had spent the day together at a conference, had a leisurely dinner, and then walked back to the garage where they were both parked a short distance from one another. They said their goodbyes and were standing by their respective cars preparing to leave when a stranger appeared from around the corner, shoved a gun up under the dispatcher's chin, and demanded money. The officer froze at the sound of the commotion. There was only a split second to decide whether to run for help and safety or stay and risk death. Abandoning a friend was out of the question. The officer pulled out a gun and screamed, "Police!"— noticing how "police" sounds like "please" when you have no saliva and your mouth is dry as cotton. The robber did not move. The officer, eyes focused on the suspect's gun, took a breath, and shot the suspect through the heart. The entire event, which seemed to take hours, was over in less than two minutes. The consequences, however, would take years to resolve.

Was this just another confrontation in the daily skirmishes of urban warfare? Not exactly. This is a modern tale. The dispatcher, the cop, and the suspect all were women.

I got called within hours of the shooting and arranged to see the officer the next morning. As a routine, when I get ready to meet a person who has just experienced a devastating trauma, I remember my scuba-diving days and how it is to enter an ocean I both fear and respect. I am excited at the prospect of seeing things below the surface that are ordinarily invisible, and I am prepared for surprises both beautiful and ugly. I try to not panic in a strong surge or to give up when it seems the shoreline has disappeared and I am lost in a sea of sadness and confusion. I remind myself that neither the officer nor I started this chain of events and that, alone, neither one of us can end it.

Lilly had blond hair and blue eyes. She was so soft-spoken and reserved that it was hard to imagine that she had killed a person less than 24 hours earlier. She sat on my couch, eyes welling, and gravely said, "I killed a woman, and I don't even know her name."

Hard to imagine a cop on *Law and Order* or *CSI* caring about such a lonely detail. But this was not a fictional cop. This was a real person struggling to understand why she of all people had been caught in the devil's own dilemma: Watch your friend die or kill a young stranger and live with the consequences. My task as psychologist would be to get her back on the job, minimize the damage to her from this devastating incident, and help her come to terms with what had happened.

Out in the waiting room, Jack, her fiancé, also a cop, was worrying about how to help—what to say, what not to say—and wondering why she and not he was being tested in this way. In the days to come, he would worry about the future and get angry at himself for being irritated over this disruption in their life together. He would feel left out in the attention focused on Lilly, abandoned by her preoccupation with herself and the event. Resenting her moodiness, he would snap at her and then spend hours berating himself for his lack of empathy. His moods would oscillate wildly between anger and remorse. He would feel guilty when thinking about his own needs and regretful that he had turned down an opportunity to attend the conference with her and her friend. He would wonder if he could have handled the shooting with less emotional aftermath.

I felt as though I had two clients who needed help: my official client, Lilly, who was directly traumatized by the fatal shooting;

and my unofficial client, Jack, who was vicariously traumatized through his association with Lilly. This is how it is always: Behind the primary trauma victim are the nearly invisible family members, friends, and coworkers whose lives are also deeply affected by the trauma—but for whom few services exist.

SHATTERED ILLUSIONS

Police favor the illusion that they are in control and not helpless. When people enter policing, they expect to be in control even when they encounter violence. They have no real way to anticipate the psychological impact of losing control or how it will feel to have a close brush with death or take another person's life, however justified. In fact, new officers get most of their information from television. They are in what psychologists call an adaptive state of denial: They must minimize the psychological and physical dangers of the job in order to be able to do it.

Fritz, a young officer I know, was nearly shot in the pursuit of some thieves who stole merchandise totaling $36. When he realized he had risked his life for such a paltry sum, he was very shaken. He had been in many prior pursuits and had always enjoyed the thrill of the chase. Now it occurred to him that he had been playing cops and robbers. Not until this close call did he understand that there were people out there who wanted to kill him—HIM! And with that realization, he began to worry about how easily his past pursuits could have turned violent and how future ones might.

Encountering violence on the job is often the first time officers realize that they can die and the extent to which they have been in denial about it. As this realization rips through officers' lives, it overwhelms their adaptive denial and alters their view of the world. Such changes in their worldview are common hallmarks among trauma victims.

After Lilly's shooting, she felt unsafe and out of control everywhere she went. Her dreams were filled with nightmare images of guns that failed to shoot. The former calm of her life was penetrated with fearful fantasies. Every nighttime noise or stranger in the street created great anxiety and disrupted any restful time she had alone or with Jack. She didn't think she could face a second incident in which she had to shoot someone, yet she was convinced such an incident was in her future. She began to track other officers she knew who had been involved in multiple life-and-death confrontations. Six weeks after her shooting, the first officer on the scene to help her was shot and killed in the line of duty, only months before he was scheduled to retire. He had survived several potentially lethal incidents prior to his death. It seemed to Lilly a bad sign, an omen that her shooting might not be the ultimate experience of her career.

Illusions can also be shattered by events that don't involve direct threats to an officer's personal safety. Marco's traumatic incident, for example, related more to his feelings of being helpless to save someone else than to protect himself. Marco was dispatched to the scene of a traffic accident; the details were sketchy, and all Marco knew was that a child had been hit by a motorcycle. When he arrived at the scene moments later, he saw that the child's injuries were massive. There was blood everywhere. Marco attempted CPR but was thwarted by damage to the child's head and profuse bleeding. The child died in the ambulance, with Marco at his side.

At the hospital, Marco was inconsolable and agitated, pacing the halls in tears as officials tried to locate the child's parents, who were out of town. He sat with the body all night long until the parents arrived, and he visited the family repeatedly for weeks after. He could not stop thinking about the child, and every time he drove by the accident site it was as if someone had turned on a slide projector inside his head that continuously reran gory scenes of the accident.

FROM STRESS TO TRAUMA: A BRIEF OVERVIEW

A traumatic event is an occurrence of such intensity and magnitude that it overwhelms a person's normal ability to cope—even such industrial-strength "copers" as cops, who are specially selected, hardy individuals trained to function in emergencies. A traumatic event involves death or serious injury, as well as intense fear, helplessness, or horror. Generally speaking, a traumatic incident destroys or cripples one's sense that life is predictable. There are many kinds of reactions to a traumatic event, ranging from a moderately uncomfortable response known as acute stress, critical incident stress, or traumatic stress, to a full-blown psychological disorder known as posttraumatic stress disorder, or PTSD.

Trauma is the intense end of a continuum that begins with general, everyday stress. *General stress,* which is not a subject of this book, affects everyone all the time and waxes or wanes with the hassle of everyday life.

Cumulative stress, sometimes known as burnout, is prolonged, unrelieved wear and tear that results from having more demands than a person can respond to. Over time, unrelenting cumulative stress can damage one's emotional and physical well-being. To be subjected to unrelenting stress or to cope poorly with the general stress of life is like riding around with your foot on the clutch; after a while, the clutch wears out. How long that takes depends on the condition of the clutch and how heavy your foot is.

On the other hand, *critical incident stress,* is incident-specific. You can point to what caused it. Critical incident stress generates considerable psychological and physical discomfort for a period of approximately two days to four weeks after the incident. This type of stress is an occupational hazard experienced by many emergency workers—police officers, firefighters, nurses, emergency medical technicians, and paramedics—following exposure to a traumatic event.

PTSD is a formally recognized mental disorder affecting about 15% of emergency services workers. PTSD creates major distress and long-lasting, disruptive changes in a person's life. It is produced by exposure to severe, usually life-threatening trauma and amplified by unresolved prior trauma, the organizational response, media events, and community reaction. Critical incident stress and PTSD are the subjects of this chapter.

IS TRAUMA CONTAGIOUS AND WHO CATCHES IT?

Most cops will never shoot their guns in the line of duty. In terms of job fatalities, it is far more dangerous to be a farmer, a taxi driver, a retail clerk, or a construction worker than a police officer. There are approximately 800,000 sworn officers in the United

States. In 2004, 132 of them were killed on duty. Fifty were murdered, and 82 died accidentally (Uniform Crime Report, 2004). With the exception of 2001, these grim statistics vary little from year to year and represent a statistical fraction of the total number of working cops. Still, one cop killed is one too many.

I know that cops and their families will worry about safety and danger no matter what the numbers are. Statistics offer little consolation for the risks cops face, nor do they make up for the daily sense of danger that one cop described as the unshakeable sensation that someone had painted a bull's-eye on the back of his uniform.

The professional bond that links cops everywhere makes one cop's trauma the property of all. One traumatic incident creates shock waves throughout the law enforcement community, causing cops and their families to ask, "What if it were me?"

Cops and their families hate to think of themselves as victims: A victim is someone else. Cops solve problems; they don't have them. This is one of the paradoxes of the police subculture: At times police demand to be seen as fully human, and at other times they reject that notion and hold themselves to be immune to human frailty. Immunity is one of the illusions that is lost or is temporarily out of service after a trauma.

When a traumatic event occurs, those most intimately associated and exposed to it will probably be the most disturbed by it, but those on the periphery can be affected as well. People on the periphery—witnesses, helpers, bystanders, coroners, evidence technicians, communications dispatchers, and families—are most at risk for falling through the cracks and not getting the help they need. This occurs because, in police agencies, the officers are on top. Civilian employees are often considered second-class citizens, if they are considered at all, and families frequently don't even enter the equation.

FIVE BASIC PRINCIPLES OF TRAUMA-RELATED STRESS

There are five concepts that are basic to understanding trauma.

1. *Trauma is in the eyes of the beholder.* What bothers you may not affect the person next to you. You may barely react today

to a major incident, and yet, next year, the same incident or a more minor one may cause you or your loved one great discomfort.

2. *The traumatic response is a normal response to an abnormal event.* There is a wide range of responses to trauma: There are no wrong ways to respond or formulas for reacting; neither is there a universal recipe for recovery. Everyone is different.

3. *Traumatic stress is a psychobiological event.* Even though traumatic stress can make you feel as though you're losing your mind, it is not all in your head. Trauma provokes a powerful response from your autonomic nervous system and activates the production of brain chemicals that affect emotions and behavior.

4. *What you resist persists.* Previous traumas that are unresolved or hidden have a significant influence in amplifying current traumatic events and hindering recovery.

5. *Coping styles count.* Hot reactors, perfectionists, rugged individualists with few support systems, and people with clinical depression, anxiety, or substance abuse problems are more at risk for PTSD.

The Eyes of the Beholder

If trauma rests in the eyes of the beholder, how do we identify traumatic events? Should we have a common understanding, or will "trauma," like the word "stress," become applied to so many situations that its essential meaning will be lost? Is it legitimate to claim to be "stressed out" by a bad haircut or "traumatized" by a lost promotion?

Some events, like war, rape, and torture, are almost universally regarded as traumatic. What confuses the issue is that people respond so differently to trauma because, I think, there are so many variables involved: the severity of the stress; the degree of terror experienced; the nature of injuries sustained; the amount of time to prepare; the meaning the individual places on the event; the degree to which the event was degrading, humiliating, or embarrassing; preevent levels of stress; the existence of previous traumas; preevent coping skills; variations in personality, genetic predisposition, and physical well-being; age; and social support.

Phil and Bernie offer a good example of different responses to the same circumstance. Both men emptied their weapons into a burglary suspect who had drawn a gun on them during a field interrogation. Bernie returned to work within a few weeks and had relatively minor problems adjusting; but Phil had major problems, and after one attempt to return to work, he developed full-blown PTSD. It took a year of psychotherapy for Phil to resolve his problems sufficiently to return to patrol duty.

What made a big difference for the two officers was their position in relation to the suspect: Bernie had stood behind the suspect, whereas Phil had faced him head on. In the few seconds prior to the shooting, there had been a silent exchange between Phil and the suspect, an exchange so primitive and powerful that no words were needed. As they looked into each other's eyes, Phil believed he could actually hear the suspect's last thoughts. Phil regarded this experience as so irrational that he told no one about it for months—he thought it meant he was crazy.

When he was shot, the suspect fell into the street between two cars and out of Bernie's sight. Convulsing in his own blood, he died with one eye open, looking straight at Phil. Bernie only briefly saw his bloodied body lying motionless in the dark. It was as though Phil and Bernie had been in two separate shootings with different suspects.

There are two major categories of traumatic incidents: natural disasters and human-made catastrophes. There is evidence that natural disasters (a police officer killed by lightening while directing traffic in a rainstorm) may be relatively less stressful because they are unavoidable. At the opposite end are preventable disasters, such as the death of an officer by friendly fire or the death of an innocent citizen by an officer in a questionable high-speed pursuit. Some traumatic incidents, like Hurricane Katrina, appear to be a mixture of both: a devastating natural disaster made worse by preventable failures in the planning and relief efforts.

The distinction between natural and human-made disasters is important for police officers because many of the traumatic incidents they experience are intentional, not accidental. Exposure to multiple ways in which humans intend to harm each other—rape, assault, robbery, abuse, terrorism—changes a person's view of the world, particularly that person's trust and admiration for others.

There is general agreement in law enforcement that the following events, alone or in combination, will trigger some type of psychological distress, usually temporary:

- Officer-involved shootings
- Prolonged incidents, especially when the outcome is undesirable (e.g., the helplessness of first responders to assist many victims of Hurricane Katrina or the search for victims in the rubble of the World Trade Center)
- Line-of-duty death
- Serious injury to an employee in the line of duty
- Serious injury to a civilian as the result of a police action (e.g., a pursuit)
- Serious multiple-casualty incidents and prolonged contact with the dead or injured
- Severe environmental destruction or human violence
- Gory scenes or gruesome details (e.g., the falling bodies at the World Trade Center or the recovery of body parts)
- Employee suicide
- Traumatic deaths of children and serious injuries to children
- Victims who are personally known to the responding officers
- Stressful living or working conditions (e.g., during the response to Hurricane Katrina, rescue personnel had no food, clothes, gasoline, batteries, or communications; 80% of the local officers were homeless; many didn't know the whereabouts of their families)
- Exposure to toxic contamination or bioterrorism, especially the presence of unknown substances

In addition, incidents that attract heavy media attention are inherently more stressful than otherwise, even though they may not be life threatening, lethal, or horrific. The same is true for actions that are later challenged or questioned (see Chapter 4).

Normal Reactions to an Abnormal Event

The signs and symptoms of a traumatic response can occur in four areas: our emotional and spiritual life, our physical well-being, our behavior, and our cognitive (intellectual) functioning. Because everyone is different, the range of signs and symptoms is highly variable.

Emotional signs of critical incident stress
- Irritability/anger/increased aggression
- Overreaction to relatively minor events
- Underreaction to provocative events
- Lack of tolerance for emotions: a tendency to experience emotions as physical states
- Preoccupation with the event and one's role in it
- Depression/suicidal thoughts
- Guilt
- Anxiety
- Emotional numbing or shock
- Loss of faith in God

Physical signs of critical incident stress
- Stomach problems/indigestion
- Headaches
- Chest pain/difficulty breathing
- Elevated blood pressure
- Hyperalertness/easily startled
- Changes in sex drive or performance
- Lots of medical problems with no diagnosable medical cause
- Dizzy spells
- Excessive trembling
- Profuse sweating

Behavioral signs of critical incident stress
- Impulsiveness/excessive risk taking/recklessness
- Silence/withdrawal/avoidance
- Problems sleeping/nightmares
- Changes in personal habits or work habits
- Changes in eating or use of drugs/alcohol
- Compulsive revisiting of circumstances resembling the initial trauma

Cognitive signs of critical incident stress

- Difficulty making decisions
- Poor concentration
- Memory problems
- Difficulty with details
- Confusion
- Difficulty in mental tasks such as mathematical calculations or report writing

Here are examples of how some unresolved or untreated signs and symptoms on these lists can show up at work.

Avoidance

Irv was working as a dispatcher in a small, rural agency. He took a domestic violence call and dispatched his close friend Charlie. Charlie's wife was riding with Charlie that day. As Charlie pulled up to the house, the abusive husband rushed outside with a shotgun. He and Charlie fired at each other, and in a minute, both lay dead in the driveway.

For months afterward, Irv responded to every domestic violence call with a curt dismissal: "This isn't a social service agency," he said; "if you have family problems, call a psychiatrist." When someone finally noticed his strange behavior, he was referred for counseling. Irv told his counselor he felt responsible for Charlie's death. He reasoned that Charlie would be alive today if he hadn't dispatched him to that call, and he wasn't ever going to put another police officer in harm's way again. So he avoided dealing with domestic violence calls. It took years of counseling for Irv to get over this tragic event.

Hyperalertness and Aggression

Rocky was so hyperalert after a shooting incident that he wore two or more guns most of the time. He even carried a gun when he took his small children swimming at their community pool. He began carrying an ankle holster, as well as his duty gun, and he was so anxious about safety that he drew his gun even on barking-dog calls. On occasion, he found himself roughing up suspects, and he once slapped a man who was in handcuffs because the man spit on him and cursed his mother. Rocky had never before been so aggressive. In fact, he had always tried to avoid working with officers he thought were too badge-heavy.

Flashbacks

Officers can respond physically to events that resemble or symbolize an aspect of the original critical incident. That's what happened to Phil. He was eager to "get back on the horse" and return to his normal life after he and Bernie killed the burglary suspect. Phil was concerned about what his coworkers were thinking about him, and he believed his prolonged absence created staffing problems in an already short-staffed department. As luck would have it, on his first night back, Phil made a felony car stop, and all the suspects in the vehicle resembled, in terms of race and clothing, the man he and his partner had killed. When Phil sighted down his gun as he had prior to the shooting, he had a flashback and saw the dead suspect's face superimposed on the current suspect. He was able to maintain the scene until help arrived, and then he fled in a panic, shaking and sweating profusely. He returned to the station, changed into street clothes, and went home. He was unable to return to work for many months and was diagnosed with chronic PTSD.

Irritability and Anger

Both of these emotions can easily lead to unprovoked quarrelsome behavior, defensiveness, and hypersensitivity to criticism or direction from colleagues or citizens, often resulting in an increase in citizens' complaints or disciplinary actions. This was Lilly's experience. Following her shooting, Lilly was angry and hypersensitive. She criticized everything and everyone around her. She bypassed the chain of command over a matter of department policy. This created a political embarrassment for her superiors and made her a troublemaker in other people's eyes. She was unable to differentiate between big and small slights. Every negative interaction created an angry response in her. She said later it was as though all the anger from the woman she killed had transferred to her at the moment of death.

Increased Alcohol Use and Altered Alcohol-Induced Behavior

Sometimes an officer who normally goes home after work starts hanging out at "choir practice," getting drunk, and behaving differently than he used to before a traumatic incident. This was the case with an officer who witnessed the accidental injury of another cop. The nature of the injured cop's wound and the sounds of his screaming in pain brought back vivid wartime memories for the witnessing officer, which he silenced with alcohol. Unfortunately, he got drunk in public and received a disciplinary action as a result.

Preoccupation with the Incident

Sara was part of a hostage-negotiating team that had a six-hour standoff with a suicidal man who ultimately killed his family and then himself. Sara couldn't stop talking about the episode. She went back to the scene again and again, listened to the dispatch tapes and telephone tapes over and over, and read and reread the clinical and investigative reports, all the while persistently Monday-morning quarterbacking herself and the rest of the team. Long after everyone else had sorrowfully moved on, Sara continued to chew on this tragedy like a dog with a bone. She couldn't talk about her profound distress at not being able to save the family; nor could she confront how terrified she was that she would get a similar call.

Certainly some preoccupation and revisiting of a critical event are associated with the psychobiology of trauma, and some review of an extraordinary incident is required to learn from it. But a great deal of the ruthless Monday-morning quarterbacking that cops do to themselves and each other is not to learn from past experience but to ward off the void of grief and helplessness that follows all loss and much trauma.

It's Not All in Your Head!: The Psychobiology of Trauma

Traumatic stress is a paradox. Because it is a *psychobiological* response, the traumatized person may be emotionally constricted at the same time his or her body is overactive—"dieseling at the curb," very much like a diesel engine that chokes and sputters long after the ignition has been turned off.

Critical incident stress and PTSD show how inseparable are our psychological and physiological reactions. Traumatic events activate hundreds, perhaps thousands, of neurological and biochemical changes. Thereafter, little things can trigger the body to react as though there were a continuing assault on one's survival and one must gear up for action.

People who are still "dieseling" seem to have poor tolerance for any kind of physical or emotional arousal and respond in an all-or-nothing way: getting very angry and hyperactive or withdrawing socially and emotionally in an effort to avoid future assaults on their nervous systems. This cycling is often unpredictable and hard on the family. Plus, a hair-trigger response can impel trauma victims to self-medicate with drugs and alcohol in order to mellow out.

The biochemistry of trauma is evident in your sense of smell, which so easily brings up old memories. The smell of forsythia instantly transports me back to my childhood summers in upstate New York. So an officer, investigating a gruesome homicide in an apartment next door to where someone is baking cookies, may long afterward see the grisly details of that crime scene whenever the scent of baking cookies is in the air. A veteran cop once told me he could remember the smell of every dead body he had encountered in his 17-year career!

In some individuals, extreme stress draws upon the body's own natural tranquilizers, the same chemicals that are supposedly responsible for runner's high. Some of these people develop an addiction to these opiates or to their own adrenalin and constantly seek to restimulate themselves. This may be why some cops come home from work and immerse themselves in newspapers, crime shows on television, and detective novels.

Since the days of the saber-toothed tiger, our bodies have been crafted to respond to threats with an assembly of physical and biochemical changes called the *fight–flight response*, although recent studies suggest that women may have a different biochemical stress response that scientists call "tend and befriend." In the fight–flight reaction, adrenal glands begin to pump adrenalin or noradrenalin. Adrenalin creates a state of biological hyperalertness. Your heart rate, blood pressure, muscle tension, and blood-sugar level all increase. Your pupils dilate. The hair stands up on the back of your arms and neck, much the way a cat's fur stands up in a fight. The blood flow to your arms and legs decreases as your neuromuscular nervous system is activated, and you get ready to run. Digestion slows down because it is a less important process than preparing to fight or flee. Respiration speeds up to provide increased oxygen, and that increased oxygen sharpens the acuteness of your five senses and further heightens alertness. Your amplified senses provide your brain with vivid sensory data with which to evaluate the situation.

The majority of officers involved in shootings report some form of distortion in one or more of their five senses. Time speeds up or slows down. What took seconds felt like hours. Sounds can be amplified or muffled. A SWAT team involved in a shooting in close quarters reported that the rounds they exchanged with the suspect sounded like cap guns, yet these guns are so loud that the officers are required to wear hearing protectors during range practice.

Visual distortions are universal. Nighttime scenes seem brightly lit, probably because of dilated pupils. Tunnel vision, the loss of peripheral sight, is common. Phil experienced such extreme tunnel vision after he shot the burglary suspect that he had to turn his whole body to see the person standing next to him. When adrenal glands pump the chemical noradrenalin, officers may feel paralyzed and unable to think. Or they may disassociate from the scene and have the sensation that they are watching themselves in a movie. This is a primitive, involuntary strategy similar to the strategy some animals use when they play dead. It is also the one remaining strategy when you can neither fight nor flee. The after-effects of this particular response, however, can have catastrophic consequences for a police officer, who may suffer from shame at having frozen rather than taken action. Disassociation can slow recovery and is a risk factor for PTSD because a person cannot fully process a traumatic event until he or she can remember all the pieces.

Whatever the symptoms, the person who returns home after a critical incident is still experiencing multiple physiological and biochemical reactions that may take days or weeks to abate. A body under extreme stress, cumulative or acute, is a bit like the Cuyahoga River in Ohio that actually caught fire because there was so much debris clogging the waterway. It is because of this stress-manufactured "debris" in the bloodstream that people under stress are advised to avoid substances that can further alter the body's biochemical balance, such as alcohol, sugar, and caffeine. It is also why medication can sometimes restore one's biochemical balance when other methods have not been successful. Strategies for recovery and healing are discussed in Chapter 6.

What You Resist Persists!

It is the nature of trauma, as it is for grief, that similar experiences piggyback on each other. The past amplifies the present. The echoes of prior experiences, particularly those that are secret, forcibly "forgotten," or never worked through, resonate with current events by magnifying them. It is as if the old issues use this new opportunity to demand relief: "Pay attention to me; pay attention to me!" they cry. This creates a double whammy, the impact of which mystifies family and friends and, most often, the affected officer, who is more surprised than anyone to be bitten by something thought long ago put to rest.

This is not to say that the officer has done anything wrong. He or she has most likely followed the common cultural wisdom that tells us not to cry over spilled milk. Most of our old hurts and memories stay comfortably tucked away in our minds. It is when something extraordinary happens—like a traumatic incident or a grievous loss—that they tumble out of the closet, begging for our attention.

Despite good training and officer safety, luck played so large a role for Fritz, the young officer who nearly got shot over $36 but survived the shooting unhurt, that it made him feel helpless and revived memories of how helpless he had felt as a child, living with a violent and unpredictable alcoholic father. He and his mother had colluded in denying that anything was wrong. "That's what fathers did on pay day: They came home drunk and threw things around. There was nothing to be upset about; you and your mother just arranged to be somewhere else on all the Fridays of your childhood," he told me.

And that's how Fritz first responded to the shooting. He suppressed his reactions. He was fine, just fine. He wasn't angry, just as he had never been angry at his father. He was tough; it didn't bother him. And then Fritz began to develop symptoms—he became frightened on the street, reluctant to chase crooks. Normally easy and outgoing, he grew irritable and began provoking civilians into confrontations so that he could release tension by getting into a fight. He became preoccupied with work, whereas before the shooting he would have left work behind after his shift ended. He began to have fantasies about getting injured on the job so he could stay home. He started avoiding his parents.

Fritz returned to see me several months after his shooting, greatly disturbed that the job he loved had become unbearable. We began to look at how his personal history was influencing his current behavior. After several months of conversations, he realized that he was still trying to be the tough-guy son his mother and father needed. He had to admit to himself that he disliked the confrontational parts of police work and never had fit that mold, although he was well regarded for his temperament and verbal skills. He hated the conformity required of cops and really wanted to do something more artistic with his life.

Ultimately he did. Had he not been in a shooting, Fritz might still be running against the grain of his own life. Although the shooting itself was not devastating, its psychological influence was intensified by Fritz's childhood and the way he had learned to cope with adversity. But because his childhood experiences and his relationship to his parents were a secret, other people thought he was faking it, exaggerating his symptoms and trying to bilk the system. Even he occasionally thought so.

Prior trauma, poor coping skills, and poor parenting don't guarantee psychological problems, but I believe they tip the percentages toward being at risk for significant levels of cumulative and acute on-the-job stress. Fritz's story is not all that unusual. Many people in various helping professions come from families in which a parent was brutal, alcoholic, or absent, or there was some other factor that made home life unpredictable. In law enforcement, a significant percentage of officers come from a home in which one parent, often the father, was dysfunctional, usually because of alcohol abuse. The officer frequently had assumed a responsible, prematurely adult role in keeping the family going. Take an informal survey yourself. While my observations are anecdotal, they are shared by many other police psychologists.

If this kind of personal history is common to the police, then many officers have learned early in life that authority figures are inherently unreliable or even destructive, a factor that might figure into the eternal and seemingly irresolvable struggles between line-level officers and management. It would also mean that many officers functioned as adults at a young age and have a brittle, perhaps unrealistic need to establish the financial or emotional security they did not have earlier in life. They may be drawn to professions that project the strong family image they never had. Their selection of a police career may be an effort to gain mastery over uncontrollable elements in their personal environment and in their psyche. When this control is shattered or the illusion of control is lost through exposure to trauma, the ramifications go deep, and old experiences and emotions are stirred up. It is a paradox that those early life experiences that may lead a person to choose police work as a career might be the very elements that undermine it.

Coping Styles Count

These days, trauma specialists prefer to talk about *risk factors* when considering why some first responders will develop PTSD and others will not. In other words, how a police officer copes with daily life before the trauma counts a lot toward how he or she will cope afterward. Researchers are still examining risk factors and looking at the impact of traumatic events on emergency personnel, and it will be years before their work is finished. But there are some preliminary findings that are useful for families to know, which I've incorporated throughout this book. For example, psychologists studying PTSD in a sample of several hundred New York City police officers before 9/11 went back and reexamined these same officers after the attack on the World Trade Center, trying to distinguish why some developed PTSD after 9/11 and some did not. What they found was that officers who experienced greater dissociation and emotional distress during the incident and had greater negative life events and less social support afterward, were the most at risk.

The benefit of identifying risk factors is that it allows mental health professionals, families, and peers to direct counseling and other services to those who are most at risk and most likely to need help. It also suggests that screening people at risk may be a better approach than forcing services on those who don't need them. Ordinary people are tougher than we give them credit for, and cops are tougher still. Most of us handle crises by doing what comes naturally: talking to friends, religious advisors, coworkers, and family members because the people who know us the best are in the best position to know what we need and when we need it.

The people who may be at a higher risk for developing PTSD, and who we therefore want to pay close attention to after a traumatic incident, are those with the following risk factors:

- Is a "hot reactor" who cannot tolerate even minor frustrations
- Has current or past problems with depression, anxiety, or major life stressors including physical illness
- Has a history of childhood abuse or other traumatic exposures
- Is a loner or rugged individualist with few support systems
- Is a perfectionist
- Has high levels of job dissatisfaction or on-the-job discrimination
- Has current or past problems with substance abuse
- Experiences terror, dissociation, or panic during the incident

POSTTRAUMATIC STRESS DISORDER

When does critical incident stress become posttraumatic stress disorder, the formally classified mental disorder? How do you know when your loved one is experiencing a universal, though uncomfortable, critical incident stress response, as opposed to full-blown PTSD, which requires professional assistance?

Mental health professionals continue to debate the definition and diagnosis of PTSD. As I understand it, some want to include a list of risk factors along with the list of symptoms and a precipitating event. Currently, the diagnosis of PTSD has certain features that never vary, despite differences in age, personality, coping skills, or community support. PTSD, acute or delayed, must follow exposure, either directly or as a witness, to an extreme trauma involving real or threatened death or serious injury. The person's response must include intense emotions of fear, helplessness, or horror that *last more than one month* and cause *significant* distress or impairment at work, at home, or in other important areas of social functioning. Generally speaking, symptoms will appear within three months of the traumatic event. While most people recover after several months, chronic symptoms can last more than a year and be triggered by cues in the environment, such as an anniversary date, a similar incident, a familiar smell, and so on.

A person with PTSD must experience one or more aspects of *each of the following three* clusters of symptoms: He or she must (1) involuntarily *reexperience* the event, (2) exhibit *avoidance or numbing* behavior, and (3) show persistent signs of *increased physical arousal*.

Signs of reexperiencing the event

- Recurrent intrusive and distressing recollections of the event; the person feels as though he or she cannot turn memories of the incident on or off at will
- Recurrent distressing dreams of the event
- Flashbacks: acting or feeling as if the traumatic event were happening again; these can occur when a person is sober or intoxicated
- Intense psychological distress over situations, sounds, or smells, and so on that symbolize or resemble an aspect of the traumatic event
- Intense nervous system activity (an adrenalin rush, profuse sweating, or rapid heart beat), upon exposure to things that resemble or symbolize the event, as though there existed a continuing threat to safety

Signs of numbing or avoidance behavior

- Efforts to avoid thoughts, feelings, or conversations associated with the trauma
- Efforts to avoid activities, places, or people that create memories of the trauma
- The inability to recall an important aspect of the trauma (this can complicate cooperating with a postincident investigation)
- Markedly diminished interest or participation in significant activities
- Feeling detached or estranged from others
- An inability to express feelings
- The sense of a foreshortened future (doubt about the success of a career, marriage, children, or a normal lifespan)

Signs of increased arousal

- Difficulty falling or staying asleep
- Irritability or outbursts of anger
- Difficulty concentrating
- Hypervigilance
- An exaggerated startle response to loud noises or unexpected movements

In spite of what has been learned about risk factors, it is difficult to predict who will develop PTSD. Research in this area remains a work in progress. What we do know, according to trauma specialist Dr. Bessel van der Kolk, is that if people live in a supportive environment, if they can talk about what happened, if the trauma has not destroyed everything they love, if they have a good sense of self and a reasonable understanding of their strengths and weakness, if their past experiences have been relatively safe, and if they are not blamed for their troubles, they can recover and integrate the experience into their lives in a way that is manageable and may produce compassion and wisdom. What Dr. van der Kolk is suggesting is that there are protective factors that safeguard individuals from PTSD and may ultimately lead to a positive outcome called *posttraumatic growth*.

Protective Factors

In the years since *I Love a Cop* was first published, research in psychology has changed direction in a profound way. Instead of focusing on what causes emotional distress, many psychologists are more interested in studying *resilience*, how people are self-righting and can use social and psychological resources to ultimately bounce back from adversity. Resilience means more than merely surviving, and it is far different from those faulty notions of invulnerability, rugged individualism, and self-sufficiency that have permeated the police profession for decades.

Resilient individuals are safeguarded by protective factors, some genetic, some learned. I describe them here, along with ideas about how these protective factors can be strengthened and supported in a cop's life. I artificially separated these factors for clarity, but in real life they overlap and intertwine.

Caring, Competent Managers

Resilience can be learned. It also needs to be modeled and supported by command staff who are informed and aware of the well-being of their subordinates and can express their concerns in an effective, helpful, and timely way. Staff who are also competent in field situations and can manage incidents effectively without adding stress. Caring organizations offer accessible low- or no-cost confidential counseling, as well as information and education about stress management and self-care for officers and their families.

A Job with a Purpose

Choosing to be a cop means dedicating oneself to socially meaningful work, a unique choice in a materialistic society that seems increasingly bent on the pursuit of personal fame and fortune. Being part of something bigger than one's own personal needs blunts the impact of the negative things police officers encounter, helps them prioritize what is and isn't important in life, and instills pride for being able to function in a crisis, something few people can do.

Family Support Systems with Positive Role Models

Police officers have two families—their work family and their real family. In my opinion, they need both. Most cops prefer talking with their families and their coworkers to consulting with professionals because they don't want to be seen as weak, and they don't believe that their conversations will be confidential (see Chapter 11). And as I said earlier, they wonder whether anyone but another cop can understand them. Social support from one's colleagues buffers the impact of negative incidents and gives cops examples of what it means to struggle well with traumatic stress. While we all know officers who exert a negative influence by encouraging cops to drink or suck it up, usually far more positive role models are available. Positive role models inspire others and provide a great reality check about what's "normal" under the circumstances. They let you know how you stand relative to the rest of the group. As much as family members matter, they cannot do this in the same way unless they are cops themselves because they can't supply the necessary technical or strategic feedback. Even so, family is absolutely key. Study after study credits family support—concern, interest, empathy and so on—with minimizing the impact of traumatic events. (I'll discuss the family's role and response to trauma more in Chapter 7.)

The Ability to Manage Strong Emotions and Impulses

The capacity to remain calm under stress or to calm down quickly after a crisis can be learned. It's not just a matter of individual effort but also the result of proper training, sufficient practice, and thorough preparation. It's hard to be calm emotionally until you are first calm physically. Some fortunate people are born with a neurological system that isn't easily ruffled. The rest of us can learn by studying deep-breathing techniques, yoga, progressive relaxation, or stress management.

The Ability to Reframe Thoughts and Perceptions

Thoughts and perceptions, especially our incorrect thoughts and distorted perceptions, trigger our emotional reactions, influence our moods, affect our behavior, and shape our physical reactions. Reframing is the ability to see something that has happened from a new and different point of view. I'm not talking about bending the truth; I'm talking about accurately looking at what has occurred from a different angle. For instance, an officer who had to make a particularly disturbing death notification was berating himself for being helpless to console the inconsolable survivors. After talking it over with his wife and his coworkers, he was able to reframe the situation. He couldn't bring the dead person back to life, which was the only possible consolation at the time, but his calm presence had helped the desperate and distracted family in very practical ways as he assisted them in notifying relatives and arranging transportation. His efforts made a horrible situation better. When he reframed the event this way, he was able to let go of the incident and accept the fact that he did the best he could under pretty terrible circumstances.

The Ability to Be an Active Problem Solver and Communicator

Cops are action-oriented, take-charge problem solvers. That's what they do for a living. The ability to face problems directly, talk things over, and openly express feelings helps people move on after a crisis. One of the great benefits of talking things over with coworkers is that you get to compare your situation with others. Knowing how others see you and see themselves can reduce a lot of anxiety. When I meet with officers after a critical incident, they are often more worried about what others think of them and what's in store for them in the future than they are about what's just occurred.

The Ability to Distance Oneself When Appropriate

Occasionally cops ask me if I think they're calloused because they don't have a lot of feelings for the victims they meet. I tell them that they need emotional detachment to function effectively on the job. When cops start thinking about victims as people, that closes the social distance. This doesn't mean that cops don't feel compassion toward others; it's just that they can't get too close or they'll wear themselves out. Distancing is a professional tool used by all helping professionals who have contact with people in pain in order to extend their usefulness to others. It's one of those paradoxes I talked about in Chapter 2: Distancing works well on the job but not at home.

The Ability to Find the Challenge in Adversity

Resilient people are optimistic, as well as practical and realistic. Resilient cops accept strong emotions and trauma as the cost of doing business and deal with them. They value what they have over what they might want but never get: money, fame, and a more perfect world. They are confident and have a positive view of themselves. When things get tough, they can count on themselves and their families to get past the rough spots. They accept their limits gracefully even while they wish they didn't have them. In a nation gone slightly mad for the game of poker, resilient people can be said to be skilled at playing a poor hand well.

Posttraumatic Growth

In the art of Chinese calligraphy, the word "crisis" is represented as a blend of danger and opportunity. This ancient wisdom is supported by recent findings that traumatic incidents are also opportunities for growth. When you ask trauma victims what they gained from their experiences, instead of focusing solely on the negative, they report the following:

Changes in themselves
- Increased self-confidence in coping with the future—after what they have endured, they feel capable of facing just about anything
- Increased self-reliance
- A blend of feeling more vulnerable—they now know that bad things happen—and stronger for having survived

Changes in their relationships with others
- Social masks being dropped; relationships with others being deepened and more intimate as a result of talking and self-disclosure

- More compassion for the suffering of others and more connection to humanity in general

Changes in their spirituality and orientation to life
- A new set of priorities for life
- A deeper appreciation for life and the people they know
- An increased emphasis on the importance that spirituality, philosophy, or religion plays in their lives

Not every trauma victim reports positive posttraumatic changes, but so many do that a distinct pattern has emerged. This doesn't mean that emergency responders won't suffer or struggle when they go through a traumatic event or that positive gains are quickly apparent. But it does strongly suggest that there is something to be salvaged from a bad situation and that family members and professionals can help trauma victims reframe a bad situation by inquiring about positive changes.

We'll continue to explore ways to find the opportunity in crisis, and move from being a traumatized victim to a resilient survivor, in the next chapter.

CHAPTER 6

FROM VICTIM TO SURVIVOR

Working Through Trauma

> Traditions of rugged individualism and toughing it
> out leave far too many police officers socially and
> emotionally isolated . . . believing that the worst of
> all the four-letter words is "help."
> —CAROL J. JOHNSTON, *Former Executive Director,*
> *New York State Office for the Prevention*
> *of Domestic Violence*

Trauma has the power to deeply affect and change our lives, though not always for the worse. As discussed at the closing of the previous chapter, traumatic experience can sometimes lead us to discover huge reservoirs of compassion and philosophical wisdom that we never knew we possessed. Trauma forces us to contemplate the inevitability of our own death and brings us face to face with grief and helplessness. So it follows that, as we recover from trauma, we must first grieve for our losses—our lost companions, as well as our lost illusions about the world and ourselves.

The process of recovering from traumatic stress is the transformation from victim to survivor. Psychologists call this *working through,* which is an oddly aerobic description for an achievement of the heart and the head. Working through trauma can make you stronger for having incorporated a powerful event into your everyday life at the same moment it connects you deeply to others. One way or another, worked through or not, trauma has the power to transform.

THE OLD WAY AND THE NEW

Cops have traditionally treated themselves for traumatic stress with copious amounts of alcohol and war stories at an after-work ritual known as "choir practice." Choir practice marks the boundary between the "battlefront" and the homefront. Many cultures recognize the innate wisdom of shifting gears after battle in order to prepare returning soldiers for normal, everyday life.

Someone should have suggested that to Kirk, a newly married young officer, who returned home after being shot at by a fleeing felon. In the middle of the night his wife got up to go to the bathroom, and when she returned to bed, he awoke, caught sight of her in a mirror, leaped out of bed, hit the floor and rolled to "safety," taking cover behind a chair before he remembered where he was and who she was. His reactions scared them stiff.

Choir practice reduces stress because it gives cops a chance to let off steam in safe company. But it is not effective over the long haul. First, the routine use of alcohol creates problems. Second, peer pressure encourages the expression of selected emotions, those that are congruent with rugged individualism and male warrior mentality. For most cops, the need to belong and be accepted is more powerful than the need to express real feelings. Feelings that get stifled never get processed. Instead, these unexpressed emotions may break through later on, camouflaged as physical aches and pains, depression, displaced anger, and so on.

The police culture—then as now—values stereotypes of masculinity and youth. Men don't complain. If things get tough on the street, it is an occupational hazard to be borne in silence or dismissed through humor. This has been reinforced repeatedly by the fictional characters who dominate novels, television, and movies. Real police officers, males and females alike, are imprisoned by these cultural stereotypes, measuring themselves and each other by an unreal standard. There is a huge cost for colluding with those fictional portraits and treating police officers as though they were immune to the consequences of their work.

Today, most officers have the benefit of a healthier, more informed, and humane work environment. They can learn psychological techniques developed from research into stress in combat and public safety; these techniques emphasize early intervention and education. Officers and their families also have access to ongoing psychological support, both professional and peer, and, as needed, excellent medication that reduces symptoms with so few side effects the officer can usually continue to work.

NO MAGIC BULLETS

There are victims and survivors: The victim is immobilized and discouraged by the traumatic event and may carry an unrealistic sense of responsibility for what happened. A survivor draws on the catastrophe as a source of strength and takes responsibility, not for the problem, but for recovering from it and moving past fear, anger, and guilt or thoughts of revenge. I tell people, "It doesn't make much difference who pushed you down the stairs; you're stuck with the limp."

There are some essential elements in recovery that will be discussed here, but there are no magic bullets. Patience and a sustainable, comprehensive effort to address the physical, psychological, and social components of traumatic stress are required. Change, when you make it, may be slow and noticeable only in the absence of something else—the first time you realize an hour went by and you didn't think about *it,* or you went shopping with your mate and walked from the car to the store without breaking out in a cold sweat.

Resolving trauma makes me think of the famous lone cypress tree in Monterey that symbolizes the rugged coastline of northern California. The wind has blown and bent this tree into a fantastic shape, and still it grows. Recovering from trauma is similar; one bows to the relentless pressure of a strong force and learns to accommodate it for all time. Trauma survivors who have successfully recovered say the traumatic incident never entirely leaves their consciousness but is integrated into their life, becoming part of who they are. You can see how hard this recovery process must be for law enforcement professionals who generally want things clearly spelled out, with specified actions leading toward measurable results that can be obtained within a designated time frame.

GOAL POSTS OF RECOVERY

Those who resolve trauma can recall the event fully, bear the feelings associated with the memory, and then, at will, turn their minds to other matters. They are no longer stuck in the memory or living their lives as if nothing but the trauma mattered. They can manage their physical state of arousal to tolerate both ordinary and extraordinary happenings with appropriate intensity. They can handle the ups and downs of intimate relationships without overreacting or withdrawing. They no longer organize their lives or their families' lives to avoid traumatic memories or feelings—like the officer who was so terrified of strangers after a shooting that he was afraid to take his family into a crowd, which meant they all had to do without ballgames, shopping malls, and movies.

Trauma survivors have restored a realistic sense of competency and self-esteem and no longer feel helpless. Any residual wariness they feel is in the service of reasonable caution. They can make long-term plans and are optimistic about the future. They are again involved in meaningful work and recreation. They have words for that which was previously unspeakable. They are prepared for relapses and know that their sense of safety may be temporarily disturbed or at the least tilted on anniversary dates or by some significant reminder of the event.

THE ROAD TO RECOVERY

The road to recovery occurs in two general phases: stabilization and working through.

Stabilization

The first thing officers have to do is feel safe and in control of their environment and the physical functions of sleeping, eating, hyperactivity, and intrusive thoughts. Ultimately, they must learn to maintain that control when faced with emotional or visual triggers that remind them of the original traumatic incident.

In the immediate aftermath of a traumatic event, not everyone appears emotionally distressed. This can be deceiving. Some officers seem numb and detached—staring off into space. These cops may be in shock and haven't had time to absorb what has happened. If you ask them how they are, they will usually reply, "Just fine," because they are so psychologically numb or exhausted they feel little else.

It is also common for people to be in denial. They may deny that a traumatic event has occurred, or they may deny the impact of their loss. This is what happened to Coleen, when her son, Mitch, was killed in the line of duty while still a rookie. At first, Coleen believed that Mitch wasn't really dead but had been given a prestigious undercover assignment and his murder and funeral faked so that he could establish a new identity. It took her nearly a year to give up this fantasy and accept his death. However painful, that acceptance marked the beginning of a long period of healing because you can't process what you can't admit.

A number of options are available to help officers stabilize after a traumatic event.

Consider Attending Critical Incident Debriefings

In the decade since I wrote *I Love a Cop*, there has been a lot of progress and controversy in the search for effective treatments for emergency personnel who develop PTSD. At the center of the controversy is the efficacy of critical incident stress debriefings. Debriefings are structured one-on-one or group conversations, often compulsory, that are scheduled for emergency responders within 24–48 hours following a significant incident. The purpose of a debriefing is to give cops an opportunity to vent, to get back in touch with others who were there, to express their appreciation for each other, to establish a sense of normalcy, and to encourage positive coping by providing information about traumatic reactions and managing critical incident stress. Family debriefings, which are held for family members only, have a similar purpose, with the added goal of providing information about traumatic stress that will help keep the lines of communication open between family members.

What has come into question in recent years is the science behind debriefings, the claims made for their effectiveness, and the unwarranted predictions that everyone who is exposed to a highly stressful situation will inevitably have future problems. Telling people about symptoms may actually make some more likely to experience the symptoms about which they've been warned. Several studies assert that debriefings have no effect on relieving or preventing PTSD, and others suggest they may actually damage at-risk participants, leaving them worse off than if they had received no intervention at all. Counseling, delivered too soon, may be too painful. Critics contend that people, especially first responders, are resilient, hardy individuals who will bounce back from adversity by using their own resources rather than depending on professionals or outsiders. What most people need after a crisis is practical, not emotional, support. For example, officers involved in responding to Hurricane Katrina were more focused on meeting basic survival needs for themselves and their families than they were in attending to their emotional needs. A better strategy, some suggest, would be to wait six to eight weeks after a crisis and then evaluate the needs of those who were directly affected or known to be at risk for PTSD.

The debate about debriefings will no doubt continue. It is hard to study debriefings because there is a lack of uniformity in how and when they are conducted, who facilitates them, who attends them, and under what conditions they are held. To further complicate matters, people who participate in debriefings often have very positive feelings about their experiences and feel empowered by information, learned skills, and support.

Until the debate is resolved, the International Society for Traumatic Stress Studies (ISTSS) recommends that participation in debriefings be voluntary; that all providers be experienced, well-trained practitioners; that debriefings focus on screening, education and support rather than on the details of the incident; that potential participants be evaluated by a trained practitioner prior to debriefing; and that further research be conducted to compare debriefings with alternative early interventions.

Take Time Off from Work

Some departments mandate that officers take a few days to a few weeks off from work following a critical incident, particularly a shooting. The amount of time off ideally should be a compromise between the officer's needs and department policy. Unfortunately, in some departments, the unplanned absence of even one officer greatly affects staffing and service.

Most officers want to rest, to connect with their families, to do something "normal." On the other hand, some individuals have an overwhelming need to be with their coworkers after a traumatic incident, and while not officially working, they may be at the station just to be part of the group. This can cause family members to feel left out and hurt.

Accept Light Duty if Needed

Some departments offer light duty assignments to injured officers. Officers who stay home for a protracted period of time may get depressed, feel isolated, and create stress for their families, so it is best for cops to get back to work as soon as it is medically and psychologically possible.

Sometimes officers with a psychological injury hate light duty work, especially at the front desk. They may be too hypertense to sit for long periods of time and too irritable to deal well with the myriad concerns and complaints that find their way to the front desks of police departments. The best light duty assignment is one that involves meaningful work and suits the officer's talents and current psychological state.

When Stanley returned to work after his shooting, he was assigned to the fleet pool, which was ideal for him because he had mechanical aptitude, was too antsy to sit still, and could justify that what he was doing served a useful purpose for his fellow officers.

John, who was injured in a bar fight, had a less than ideal assignment. He was placed at the front desk because there was no other light duty work available. He was short-tempered with citizens, was distracted, and finally had to be relieved from duty after ripping the phone from the desk because it rang too often.

Get Accurate Information and Feedback

It is really important for officers to get accurate information about their incident. I cannot emphasize this point too strongly. Research has demonstrated that accurate information is a powerful antidote to anxiety, especially after a critical event.

Remember Phil. Phil was the officer who had a harder time recovering from his shooting than his partner, Bernie. Immediately after the shooting, Phil was terrified that someone would kick the suspect's gun away, and it would appear that the shooting was unjustified. He stood pointing his weapon at the suspect's gun until another cop literally moved him off that spot and uncurled his fingers from his gun. He needed to know that he was safe, that the threat was gone, and that he had done the right thing.

Both Phil and Bernie required accurate, immediate, and ongoing information about the legality of the shooting and the progress of the investigation in order to manage their concerns about lawsuits, discipline, and job security. They also needed information about traumatic stress reactions—what is considered normal, how long it goes on, how to cope, and when to yell for help. They got the psychological information during a debriefing.

Consider Taking Medication

Medication may provide relief for people whose physical symptoms are persistent or extreme, although it is very important that they agree to take medication, lest they again feel out of control of their own destinies. Medication can be used to "reset" the nervous system. There are many kinds of psychoactive medications that affect various components of the nervous system—far too many to discuss here. Clinical reports have claimed success for nearly every class of medication. For acute stress, it's important to interrupt the body's continued outpouring of stress-related hormones by seeking help as soon after the incident as possible, especially for officers whose resting heart rates are above 90 beats per minute, who have experienced dissociative reactions (feelings of unreality or an inability to recall an important part of the event), or have endured moments of extreme terror.

I recommend consulting a psychiatrist for medication. Although it is perhaps easier to have your familiar and accessible internist prescribe something, most psychiatrists stay on top of the frequent new developments in psychoactive medication in a way that internists, who are generalists, cannot. I know that the stigma attached to seeing a psychiatrist may be a big hurdle, but think of it this way: You wouldn't want your dentist to remove your appendix, even if your dentist is top-notch in his or her field. (See Chapter 11 for suggestions about choosing a therapist.)

It is also important to have patience. Some psychoactive drugs take time to kick in, and the dose may need to be adjusted several times to suit the individual. In the case of extreme anxiety or discomfort, a psychiatrist can temporarily prescribe faster-acting medication to tide the patient over until the primary medication takes effect.

Obtain Psychological Support

There are many forms of psychological support specifically designed to deal with the discomfort of critical incident stress or PTSD. Among these are cognitive-behavioral therapy, psychotherapy, peer support, stress management, biofeedback, meditation, hypnosis, and eye movement densensitization and reprocessing.

Cognitive-behavioral therapy (CBT) is probably the most promising, effective, well-documented approach to treating incident-specific trauma. It consists of a short series of highly structured individual appointments with a specifically trained therapist, each lasting from 60 to 90 minutes. During these sessions, clients are educated about traumatic reactions, taught progressive muscle relaxation, systematically exposed to visual memories of the traumatic incident, helped to restructure beliefs they may hold about themselves or the incident, and gradually reintroduced to situations they may be avoiding. Clients are active participants in the therapy and will be required to do a bit of homework between sessions, such as monitoring their feelings, actions, and thoughts.

Psychotherapy is more broadly focused. The therapist is interested in your childhood, your family of origin, and other dimensions of your current life beyond the traumatic incident. People at risk for PTSD often struggle concurrently with other long-standing psychological conditions such as anxiety, depression, or childhood abuse. If your loved one's postincident symptoms don't abate within 30 days, consider seeking psychological help from a therapist trained in CBT. If he or she has had problems prior to the incident, be sure to tell the CBT therapist and ask for a referral to a general therapist once CBT treatment has concluded. Is it always beneficial to work with a police psychologist? Probably so if your presenting problems have something to do with your work. (See Chapter 11, "Getting the Help You Need When You Need It.")

Peer support is based on the notion that an officer is most likely to confide in someone he or she trusts and knows rather than turn to a stranger. It is also based on the idea that officers have walked in each other's shoes and can understand, perhaps faster and better than family or friends, what a cop goes through. One of the most powerful sources of psychological support comes from one's peers. Peer supporters are trained in listening skills and crisis intervention. They are taught to recognize the signs and symptoms of serious problems and know when and how to refer someone for professional help. They may assist mental health professionals in debriefings. Very often they act as role models because they have experienced and resolved traumatic stress. Although not a substitute for professional mental health care, they provide day-to-day, round-the-clock emotional support for their fellow officers.

Stress management is a comprehensive, skill-building program with the ultimate goal of teaching new living habits that reduce both acute and cumulative stress. A comprehensive stress management package will usually include information and training in the following areas: exercise; nutrition; the use and misuse of stimulants and alcohol; and the practice of calming techniques such as biofeedback, meditation, deep breathing, visualization, and/or progressive muscle relaxation.

Biofeedback is like a high-tech Zen. A psychologist or trained technician teaches you to control various physiological processes with the aid of monitoring devices that measure muscle tension, skin temperature, and so on. These devices give you feedback. Biofeedback technology has been successfully used to treat a variety of conditions: gastrointestinal problems, headaches, muscular–skeletal problems, high blood pressure, and general tension, to name a few.

Meditation, deep breathing, and hypnosis are immensely effective in treating critical incident stress, PTSD, and other forms of anxiety. Meditation can be as simple as the private, daily practice of taking time out to focus on your breathing. Prayer, too, has calming effects similar to meditation.

Eye movement desensitization and reprocessing (EMDR) is an experimental treatment developed in the late 1980s. It involves recalling a traumatic incident in full sensory and emotional detail while simultaneously moving one's eyes according to instructions from a therapist trained in EMDR techniques. Some trauma victims treated with EMDR report symptomatic relief, often following a single eye movement session. Many police psychologists are using EMDR in their practices, frequently in conjunction with other brief therapy interventions. EMDR may be helpful in reducing the uncomfortable symptoms associated with a traumatic event, but it may not be sufficient to manage the cumulative stress, family strain, and lifestyle issues that often accompany a police career.

Working Through

Once stabilized, your cop will begin working through the emotional aftermath of a traumatic event by finding meaning in what has happened, rewriting some core beliefs, dealing with ambivalence about the job, integrating the experience, mourning his or her losses, and then finally staking out new territory.

Finding Meaning in What Happened

Human beings seem to be wired in such a way that we cannot rest until we can make sense of our experiences. No time is this more true than after a traumatic event. Dr. Charles Figley, trauma expert, explains that the process of working through trauma requires that the victim address some fundamental questions: "What happened?" "Why did it happen?" "Why did I act as I did?" "Why do I act as I have since?" "What if it happens again?" Cops who can stay the course and contain the emotions that are generated by such questions will come out the other end significantly changed, usually for the better.

Rewriting Core Beliefs

One of the most hurtful consequences of trauma is the shattering of certain core beliefs such as the myth of indestructibility or the belief that one should always be in control. What may be left in their place is another set of core beliefs about how life is unpredictable and how helpless or inadequate the cop is to deal with life's ups and downs. Healing from trauma requires that an officer rewrite his or her original core beliefs, as well as the newer set of beliefs developed after the traumatic incident.

Following Phil's shooting and his premature and unsuccessful return to duty, much of our work together focused on rewriting those beliefs about how his worth as a human being was dependent on his performance as a cop. This had led to a system of values that placed the job before his personal relationships and before his own health. He believed that he was invincible and couldn't get hurt. (While that sounds ridiculous, it is so hard to imagine dying that we commonly harbor the secret belief that we won't, until we see our parents and friends die or face near death ourselves.) He believed anything less than perfection wasn't good enough, that he was so tough he could and should absorb unlimited amounts of stress without consequence and that he must never feel afraid.

It was our job to look at the history of those beliefs, examine what positive purpose they may have served in Phil's life, and then decide how they could be rewritten in a more realistic and manageable way. Phil, like many other officers, learned early in life to suppress his feelings and keep his problems to himself in order not to upset his parents, who were burdened by serious illness and financial difficulty. His self-reliance and emotional hardiness as a child were major contributions to the stability of his family. But without modification, these psychological habits and core beliefs were harmful to him as an adult.

Since our core beliefs about life and about ourselves are often unstated, there is no way to check to see if they are accurate or realistic. If they are not realistic or manageable, they propel us to behave in ways that are inherently stressful and create more problems. For example, the idea that I must never disappoint anyone or show any weakness or that people must always be pleased with me makes me try to achieve the impossible and leaves me certain to fail miserably. These beliefs are delivered in the form of inner chatter, or self-talk. People feel great relief when they challenge themselves to rewrite their strident beliefs and change their self-talk to a more reasonable and positive tone.

Dealing with Ambivalence

Officers quite naturally experience great ambivalence about returning to work after a traumatic incident. They have ongoing safety concerns and are usually apprehensive about how they will act in the future if faced with a similar threat.

Tackling ambivalence involves answering some of those hard questions mentioned above. This was the case with Chris, who came to my office after an encounter with a senior citizen who stuck a fake gun in his chest after Chris had responded to a silent alarm at a senior citizens' center. I had worked with Chris before as he had experienced other frightening and dangerous encounters. He was furious with himself for letting his guard down and assuming that the well-dressed, elderly man was no threat. He was badly shaken by a litany of what-ifs—what if the gun had been real? What if he had shot or been shot? What if he had lost control and hit this old guy? He was second-guessing himself all over the place and wondering if he should continue as a cop. His confidence was low, and he was depressed because he felt asking for my assistance again meant he was backsliding.

To the contrary, I thought his asking for help in a timely manner, rather than toughing it out alone as he had before, was an indication that he was dealing better with stress. It was obvious that these close calls were mounting up, and he was worried that the probability of his getting seriously hurt one day was increasing. He was also afraid he might overreact to his next man-with-a-gun encounter and shoot prematurely. As before, Chris had hidden this incident from his family, although he worried about them and how they would handle his being shot in the line of duty. He imagined them driving by and seeing his body lying in the street.

I encouraged Chris to go home and tell his wife what happened. When he returned the next week, he felt much better because of this talk. We could both see a pattern: What he resisted persisted. The more he talked, the better he felt. Sharing this incident with his wife helped him to feel less guilty about loving a dangerous profession that entailed risk and potential loss for his family and his children. His wife was able to tell him that she was more upset by the emotional distance he created by keeping things to himself than the less likely probability that he would be killed in the line of duty.

Chris's ambivalence about returning to work is a common response to traumatic stress and one that creates anxiety for both officer and family, who depend on the job for financial security. This is a time when the best course of action may not be obvious. Cops may be caught between a rock and a hard place: Either return to work—a place now fraught with danger and bad memories—or file a stress claim and throw themselves on the mercy of a system that is adversarial, hostile, and indifferent. The third alternative is to cut their losses and walk away from a career and a retirement package. The best advice is to make no important decisions while at the beginning stage of resolution: Take some time off; get some counseling.

Integrating the Experience

Contrary to what you might think at first, successfully working through trauma means that you integrate, not exorcise, the traumatic memory. For weeks and months, your cop may be cycling between closing off emotionally and falling victim to floods of emotion associated with unwanted memories or reminders of the event. He or she may refuse to discuss the event in order to avoid the emotions attached to it.

To integrate a traumatic event, most people need to reclaim full memory of the incident and all the associated emotions. However, it is important that your officer has full say over the pace of his or her recollections and sufficient time to reestablish emotional control once it is lost. For this reason, therapy sessions with a traumatized cop can rarely be handled in the traditional 50-minute hour, especially at the beginning of treatment.

Even though talking to another person is still the primary outlet for working through trauma, people are helped by writing in journals, expressing themselves through artistic means, joining self-help groups, or giving testimony about their experiences in an effort to help others. Again, the important thing is that the officer makes the choice.

It took Lilly over a year to integrate what had happened to her. For months she dreamed of bodies that wouldn't stay buried as she fought against thinking about the shooting. She had to reconcile how she could be a daughter, a sister, a fiancée, a friend, a caring citizen, a lover of animals, and a person who had killed. She had to integrate two selves: one, a brave, feisty, and competent cop; the other, a frightened woman who panicked at the sight of a stranger on the street.

Integrating Shootings

Fatal shootings may be hard to integrate. Although precise figures aren't available, it has been reported that 50 to 80% of all officers who kill leave law enforcement within five years. My advice is to take these numbers with a grain of salt. Nobody can predict with certainty how someone else will react after a shooting. Everyone responds differently, and there is tremendous variation around the circumstances of every shooting.

Why would an officer leave his or her job after a fatal shooting? For some, the act of killing another human being, even when the shooting is justified, may create moral pain and run against the grain of an officer's most essential values. It is a myth that officers involved in legitimate killings have no problems and relish the hero worship of coworkers and the community. In many instances, the officer bears both psychological scars and social stigma. The officer who kills is the purveyor and survivor of trauma. In instances where the person killed was innocent or killed by accident, the moral pain may be unbearable.

Dick, for example, shot and killed a parolee during a nighttime drug bust. The shooting was legitimate since the parolee charged the officers and appeared to have a weapon in hand. Unfortunately, the weapon turned out to be a hair comb. Dick felt like an executioner. No amount of reassurance from his coworkers could ease his bitter self-recriminations or stop him from second-guessing his actions over and over.

Officers who have killed may feel both a mixture of relief and repulsion at having met a challenge they've been thinking about since their first day on the job. Most of us never have to face our ability to kill as did Lilly, Phil, and Dick. Killing someone alters a person's sense of him- or herself. Cops who kill may need some professional assistance to integrate the event. Their families can also profit from counseling.

On the other hand, research published in 2004 paints a more hopeful picture. Sociologist and former police officer David Klinger interviewed 80 officers and sheriff's deputies who had shot someone in the line of duty. Few officers in his study suffered any long-lasting negative effects, and nearly 30% felt elated after their shootings. They were joyful and excited at surviving life-threatening situations and proud of their abilities to use appropriate deadly force. Only 12% reported feeling guilty. Still, Dr. Klinger cautions that most shootings create a "notable disruption" immediately afterward and that long-term problems, although infrequent, are by no means rare. He endorses the benefits of peer and supervisory support—officers who lacked this support reported the most severe and long-lasting negative reactions. But he is critical of any procedure that amplifies post-shooting reactions through the power of suggestion. Dr. Klinger specifically cites some preincident training designed by mental health professionals for placing too great an emphasis on the negative and certain post-shooting protocols, such as mandatory critical incident debriefings, for presuming that officers who have been involved in shootings are destined for trouble.

Mourning

Learning to live with what happened paradoxically involves letting it go. It is hard to let go of something or someone without first mourning your loss. To mourn your loss, you must accept it. Grief and helplessness are the cornerstones of traumatic stress. We grieve for what we have lost—companions, illusions of invincibility, youthful potential, and so on. One of the diagnostic indicators of traumatic stress is loss: loss of emotions, loss of interest in significant activities and people, loss of memory, loss of an enduring sense of self, loss of a sense of safety, and loss of adaptive denial.

Grief can be unbearable and disorienting. The griever is stuck with loss and emptiness and is helpless to undo either. Cops are action-oriented problem solvers who detest feeling helpless or passive. They seek relief in activity and fantasies of revenge. Since guilt is a more active emotion than grief, I only half-jokingly suggest that cops prefer beating up on themselves to grieving because it gives them something to do!

Staking Out New Territory

Officers bring closure to their experience when they are ready to put their new core beliefs and their new view of themselves and the world to the test. They may take an active stance and fight to regain what they have lost or fight for what they have decided they need. It is at this point that some officers make the decision to leave police work, feeling they have made a contribution and now want to do something else that is more consistent with their new view of themselves and the world. They may remake an early career decision and opt for a job that allows them more autonomy or individuality. Part of their restored self-image is intolerant of any future self-sacrifice, and they may have much clearer ideas of what they want and need from their work.

In staking out new territory, cops come to know themselves and to develop compassion and forgiveness for their limitations and, consequently, for the limitations of others. They can see positive aspects of their traumatic experience while simultaneously acknowledging that these positive outcomes were won at too great a price. They are more open with others and less afraid of intimacy. Often, they are more appreciative of how much their families have suffered as a result of their preoccupation with trauma. They give up feeling special about being a cop or for having undergone a serious traumatic incident. They recognize that suffering is part of the human condition and not their own personal trial.

As cops stake out new territory, they frequently look for a way to use their personal experience to help others. This in turn helps them bring meaning and closure to their individual torment. Chris started a peer support group in his agency. Phil and Danny testified to their fellow officers in advanced officer training. Phil told about his shooting and his flashback, and Danny talked about losing a fist fight and the long sequence of physical and emotional symptoms that plagued him for years. Lilly started a self-help group for cops.

CHAPTER 7

FROM BATTLEFRONT TO HOMEFRONT

Families and Trauma

It cannot be reiterated too often:
No one can face trauma alone.
—JUDITH HERMAN, MD,
Trauma and Recovery

In 1944, World War II brides could purchase a pamphlet for 15 cents entitled "When He Comes Back and if He Comes Back Nervous." This pamphlet offered a list of suggestions for dealing with the soldier but had scant advice for the wife. Spouses were urged to get professional help rather than "muddle through," and they were cryptically coaxed to "let your own faith and beauty of spirit be your chief stock in trade"—hardly concrete counseling for dealing with a disoriented, perhaps violent loved one who has returned home from war a stranger.

Although being a police officer is not the same as being at war, we've learned from the families of combat veterans and war survivors that the love and compassion of family is a potent factor in helping someone heal after a traumatic incident. But we also know that trauma is contagious and, like secondary smoke, can contaminate family life. And we've seen that love and compassion, which are the family's strength, can also be its Achilles heel.

If traumatic stress strikes your family, you'll need to think about what you can do to help your mate or your friend, what you can do to help yourself, and what you can do to assist your children.

HELPING YOUR MATE

Although families can do a lot to help an officer recover from trauma, the bottom line is that no matter how much you love someone, you cannot dissolve that person's trauma nor recuperate for him or her. What you can do is manage the consequences in order to minimize the impact on yourself and your family. You can avoid creating a second injury, and you can try to go on as normally as possible. The first thing to do is what you are doing right now: learning about trauma and traumatic reactions. I encourage you to reread the sections in Chapter 5 that discuss critical incident stress, PTSD, and the ways in which coping styles and other protective factors can help reduce the risk for developing posttraumatic stress. Armed with that overview, you'll be better equipped to understand the impact of trauma on the family and the family's role in helping the officer work through trauma.

Acknowledging Something Is Wrong

Families are true first responders and often know well before supervisors and friends that something is wrong even if the cop doesn't spell it out. You may not know what's troubling your mate, but your intimate knowledge of his or her behavior leads you to spot those subtle changes that indicate something is out of order: problems sleeping, a change in appetite or mood, and so on. Because you have an early warning system, you can confront your loved one and urge that he or she talk about what is wrong or seek professional help.

For example, after Woody was shot, his mood was euphoric. He had survived and had done so because he was mentally well prepared. He was receiving lots of attention and positive acclaim. His injuries were relatively minor. Within days, he and his brother had a huge fight that stopped short of coming to blows. His mother observed that Woody had a very short fuse and was far too angry over a minor miscommunication with his brother.

Woody's mother did something very wise. She insisted Woody get professional help and that the whole family meet with a therapist so they could understand what was happening and how they could help. She also set her bottom line on what was acceptable behavior. She told Woody in no uncertain terms that she did not like his angry outbursts and would not tolerate them.

Her reactions encouraged Woody to get the help he needed early on and also gave him a reality check that prompted him to get back in control of his emotions and his behavior. When he did so, he felt much better. His mother didn't yell at him, argue with him, or plead, but she presented her ideas calmly and confidently. She was the epitome of the old adage: "gentle pressure, relentlessly applied." Had Woody refused her suggestions, she would have sought help for herself and the rest of the family. Professional help is in order if your cop

- Is experiencing severe mood swings
- Can't sleep for days
- Has repeated nightmares
- Has angry or violent outbursts
- Is depressed, guilt-ridden, or suicidal
- Uses alcohol or other drugs to excess
- Is not back to normal after four weeks

Reassurance

Because you have a history together, you can help blunt the overly negative self-appraisal that often follows traumatic stress. If you try to talk someone out of his or her feelings, you risk making that person feel as though you don't understand. Still, you can remind your officer that one sin is *not* worth a thousand good deeds and then point to the usually long list of kind acts, accomplishments, and positive qualities that make him or her a respected family member and friend. You can help your mate separate his behavior from who he is as a person. You can remind her that a violent action taken at work does not mean she is a violent person. You can place blame and credit more objectively.

Friends and family can also provide reassurance by helping the officer remember how he or she successfully coped with other tough times or incidents. Remembering past successes makes a person feel less helpless or overwhelmed.

You can help your officer with these five big questions: What happened? Why did it happen? Why did I act as I did then? Why did I act as I have since? What if it happens again? You don't have to provide the answers because, by talking it through, your cop will probably come up with a response of his or her own.

You can also normalize the traumatic experience for your mate by suggesting, for example, that given what she has been through, if she weren't stressed, she wouldn't be human. In other words, you are continuously reminding your loved one that stress is a normal response to an abnormal event. This is very reassuring since traumatized cops often feel as if they're going crazy.

Witnessing

One of the most important things you can do as family member or friend is to provide witness: to listen to your cop's story without judgment. While this sounds and sometimes feels as if you're not doing much, sharing a story helps to soften an experience that is more horrible if contained in isolation. Telling one's story to an interested, empathic listener is the foundation of all the healing professions and of much religious activity, from confession to prayer.

Because traumatic incidents are often recalled in bits and pieces, patiently listening to the retelling of a personal story can bring out forgotten details and emotions that may be begging to be recalled. Your cop will find a lot of coworkers are willing to collude with him or her in covering up or pretending everything is "great, just great." Your willingness to hear the story out and tolerate the strong feelings that might go with it—when your officer is ready to tell it—is very supportive. Your cop's willingness to share it is a vote of confidence in you.

This is what happened to Greg. Early in his career he was working undercover, sitting at a table with a drug dealer to negotiate the purchase of some crack cocaine. Suddenly the bad guy pointed a gun directly at Greg and pulled the trigger. Nothing happened. The gun didn't go off, and Greg didn't flinch, though he felt as though he'd been through an earthquake. The bad guy, satisfied with his "test," pronounced Greg "cool."

Greg was elated; he had stayed the test of courage and walked tall in front of his fellow officers. It was a big feather in his cap, but he kept the experience from his wife because he didn't want to frighten her. He had always protected her from the realities of his work, and he actually believed she thought he worked at a desk most of the day.

Years later, now the father of twin boys, he repeated this story to his new brother-in-law, who is also a cop. As he was telling it, he was surprised to feel a lump in his throat. He went back home and couldn't stop thinking about the incident, about his children, and about how burned out he had been feeling since the twins were born. He then realized that he was feeling more frightened than burned out. He traced this fear back to the incident with the drug dealer, thinking concurrently how he is the whole world to his boys, that everything is "Daddy this" and "Daddy that," and how, if he were killed, his kids would be devastated. The patience with which his brother-in-law listened allowed Greg to recover the rest of his story and connect it to current difficulties in his professional life. Having done so, he felt that a big load was lifted off his shoulders, and he noticed a return of enthusiasm and interest in work.

Listening has advantages for you, as well as your officer. Giving your loved one the opportunity to express strong anger, guilt, and grief will help speed the recovery process and may make you feel closer to each other. Relish the intimacy of emotional expression that sometimes follows traumatic incidents; you may miss it when the person recovers and is back to his or her normal, less-expressive self. Phil's fiancée and Woody's family reported feeling closer to them than they had in a long time. Both men were so affected by their traumatic experiences that they were more loving, emotional, and communicative than usual. The near loss of their lives made their families more precious to them.

Pinch Hitting

All families develop roles, sometimes by design and often by accident. Those roles become solidified by habit or inertia and are reinforced by tradition. In times of crisis, family members should try to be flexible in their roles and chores, pitching in for each other in a variety of ways.

People under stress often have trouble concentrating or getting energized. Providing some concrete assistance with domestic chores can relieve an already stressed person of the strains of everyday life and keeps reassuring, normal routines in order. Offer to do laundry, go food shopping, take over paying the bills, babysit, or provide transportation to the doctor's or lawyer's office. Help with legal documents, make phone calls, or polish shoes. Take your cue from the officer.

One exception to pinch hitting pertains to children. Children can help their parents and be involved in family matters, but they should not assume an overly adult role and act like parents to their own parents, which—as I have suggested—was the childhood experience of many police officers.

The Arsenic Hour

There's an arsenic hour—when everyone has needs, and no one has anything to give—every day in many families, but especially following a traumatic incident. It adds to the stress if you and your spouse have very different expectations after a critical incident, like Sam, who after breaking up a gang fight expected open arms and a warm meal only to find that his wife had the flu and was waiting for him to come home and cook.

It is hard to predict what your cop might need or want after a critical incident. Some cops are exhausted and need to rest or sleep. Others are adrenalinized—fatigued yet too restless to slow down, jumpy, irritable, and angry with others who aren't moving or driving fast enough.

Everyone has different needs for talking. You may want to ask questions, talk about your experiences—where you were when you heard about the incident, what the kids were doing, and so on. In contrast, your mate may not want to talk because he or she is tired or still processing what happened. Some people alternate between wanting and not wanting to talk. This can drive everyone around them a little crazy.

When a cop says, "I don't care," "I don't know," or "I don't want to talk about it," it may well mean he or she is covering up feelings. It is important not to collude with a person who is covering up. On the other hand, it's not wise to force or nag a person to talk before that person is ready. Occasionally cops just get tired of repeating their story. The best thing you can do is not cover over your own feelings. Don't pretend *you* don't care when you do.

On the other hand, your cop may be supersensitive to your reactions, reading you for the slightest sign of inattention, boredom, skepticism, and so on. She may want you to feel what she feels, which is impossible. Gently remind him that you didn't live through the experience the way he did, and that while you're interested in the incident itself, you are more interested in him.

Check out your expectations and try to keep them realistic. *You* may expect to have a long, intimate talk, but your cop prefers to sleep or talk on the phone with his or her coworkers. You may have cooked a fabulous dinner as a way to show your love and concern only to find that your spouse has already eaten. Or you may accidentally cook a meal of red meat or ribs that reminds your cop of the incident—particularly if it was bloody—and he or she gets nauseated and can't sit at the table. You may feel you should have known better, when, of course, you couldn't have.

Don't be surprised if your cop cannot relate to family life because everything seems minor or trivial in comparison with what he or she has just been through or witnessed. An officer who has just seen a child cut in half by a train may have little sympathy for a scraped knee. This is temporary and not intentionally done to hurt anyone. Gently bring it to his or her attention.

YOUR ACHILLES HEEL

It is unbearable to sit by and watch someone you love suffer with emotional or physical pain. Because you love your mate, you may think you ought to be able to help or at the very least know what he or she is feeling. The natural thing to think is that if you don't, you are doing something wrong and should try harder. Because you are sensitive to this person, you can literally feel his or her pain, rage, hopelessness, or fear. Children are particularly affected by their parents' moods and the level of stress they observe. But they react even more deeply to disagreements their parents have over the traumatic event or its aftermath.

Because you are a police family, you may think you should be able to solve most problems. When you think about it, solving a problem for someone else implies that you know what's best for that individual or that he or she can't figure it out alone. Attempting to rescue another adult who is not grievously impaired is often a measure of your own discomfort and anxiety—a cue that you need some support and counsel for yourself. It is often hard to know when you are being responsive or overly responsible.

Men in our society, especially, have been conditioned to think it's their role to rescue others and provide solutions. This often sets them at odds with the women in their lives. For instance, when Megan was a new supervisor, she was involved in an undercover operation that fell apart, and an officer was injured. She was consumed with guilt and self-loathing for her "failure" to have supervised the situation better. Her department had a very negative view of her behavior and disciplined her severely.

Richard, her husband, was infuriated. He pushed her to quit, and when she wouldn't, he urged her to sue. Her distress became his distress, so much so that his feelings were at the center of most of their conversations, and Megan felt as though she was fading into the background and losing control of the situation. She felt so much pressure from Richard that she began to feel as though she was failing him, too, by not fighting back, when all she really wanted was to put the whole incident behind her and go on. Richard was so frightened by her depression he thought the only way he could help was to tell Megan what to do next. All Megan needed was for him to listen sympathetically, be patient, provide feedback when she asked for it, and not panic when she didn't respond according to his time line.

While quitting may be the best and most appropriate move for some, it is a grave decision and one that should not be made under pressure. Leaving police work can lead to a sense of failure and of being a quitter. The person may have regrets later on when he or she feels better and stronger.

I have heard cops complain about therapists they consulted after a traumatic incident. These therapists were unfamiliar with law enforcement and made a snap diagnosis that leaving police work would be the solution to their clients' problems. In every instance, this suggestion felt like an uninformed and insensitive slap in the face and was discarded, along with the therapist's services.

If you want to see your loved one in a safer, saner profession, you should talk openly about your fears, and they should be given serious consideration. However, pressuring your mate to leave police work is more apt to create resentment and defensiveness than it is to create open dialogue and respect for your concerns.

Tips for Dealing with a Cop in Crisis

- Accept that a crisis has occurred, and be prepared for the fact that it will affect your relationship. Remind yourself that it is not your fault.
- Traumatic stress may be damaging to the warmth and intimacy of family life and friendship. Accept that you might be angry about this disruption.
- Remember that trauma is in the eyes of the beholder. Even if you don't think something is traumatic, accept that your loved one does. A teenager with a broken heart feels as though the world is over, and while you know it isn't, you treat his or her broken heart with seriousness, empathy, and perspective.
- Remember this disruption is usually temporary and responds well to intervention.
- Focus on problem solving rather than assigning blame. Look toward the solution that will create a "new normal" for your life and help you move ahead.
- Traumatic incidents can bring out or exaggerate differences between people. Don't automatically assume these differences raise impossible obstacles to intimacy or that people who love each other will think alike.
- Express your commitment and affection. Sometimes the best a family can do is to say, in one way or another, "We love you, and we'll stick with you."
- Express anger appropriately. Have zero tolerance for violence. You cannot help anyone by allowing him or her to

(cont.)

(continued from previous page)

abuse you or vice versa. If violence erupts as a consequence of crisis, please see Chapter 9, "Domestic Abuse," and look in the Resources section for help.

- Avoid substance abuse. Alcohol and drugs complicate recovery and can lead to domestic violence. Children will often act out in protest when a parent is abusing drugs or alcohol. Substance abuse usually requires the help of an outside source, such as Alcoholics Anonymous, or a mental health professional. Families can find help through Al-Anon or Alateen. (See Chapter 10, "Alcohol Abuse and Suicide," and look in the Resources section for additional help.)

- Provide companionship. Being together and doing enjoyable things will help reduce the feeling of isolation. Temporary escape and distraction may remind the person that there is life beyond his or her own traumatic experience. Time spent in nature may put things into perspective.

- Fight feeling guilty. When something bad happens to someone you love, you may feel guilty for having been spared. It is a false assumption to think that your limitless dedication and devotion can ever compensate for someone else's suffering or that ignoring your own interests and needs for recreation, socialization, or comfort will hasten his or her recovery. Take as good care of yourself as you take care of others.

- Set reasonable limits. Do not let trauma hold you or your family hostage.

HELPING YOURSELF AND YOUR FAMILY

When one member of the family is in pain, all are in pain. Trauma is a family issue. Therefore, it is important to distinguish between traumatic events and the soap opera of everyday life. To some officers, a promotional opportunity is a trauma, and the whole family is expected to tiptoe around while they study.

Woody's shooting was really traumatic for him and his family. His mother felt guilty because she was a religious woman who prayed for Woody every day, and the day of his shooting she had fallen asleep without saying her prayers. His father was also upset because he usually said "good-bye" and "good luck" to Woody as he went to work, but he had been asleep when Woody left the house at the crack of dawn. Both of them needed the opportunity to talk about their feelings and get some feedback from Woody.

As a general rule, partners need to have their own support systems and not be entirely dependent on their mates for emotional consolation. This is especially true after a traumatic incident, when family members can be easy targets for a confusing array of displaced feelings. It's not atypical for an officer attending the tragic, gruesome death of a child to rush home, embrace his or her children, and then alienate them by excessively limiting their behavior in an effort to keep them safe from harm.

Try to buddy up with another police spouse or friend. You and your buddy can provide each other with reciprocal support free from the need to keep a stiff upper lip, be strong, be cheerful, and so on in front of the family. Support will help you deal with the days your loved one is moody, irritable, or preoccupied with the incident. The fact that these are normal responses to trauma doesn't make them any easier to live with.

It is healthy to interact with others—friends, family, neighbors, relatives, church members, community resources, and health professionals. Unhealthy families hide behind closed doors, and their real life is a secret. It's a mistake to assume you can handle this alone, although it's typical of law enforcement families to be so independent that they feel they are violating some deeply held value to ask for help. Maybe all you need is someone to witness your life, walk with you around the block, give you a little practical assistance, or simply listen. Emotional support is what puts gas back in your tank and provides you with perspective.

A traumatically stressed person may be very self-centered and behave as though the world revolved around his or her experience. Don't resign yourself to being left out or isolated—speak up.

This is what happened to Art's fiancée, Caroline. Several weeks after Art's closest friend was shot to death in the line of duty, Caroline suddenly burst into tears, saying she was sick of Art being so grumpy and grouchy. Caroline had a gunny sack of feelings she had been keeping to herself since the shooting because she was trying to be supportive of Art. She felt she had no right to her own feelings or needs because they paled in comparison to losing a best friend that way. Art encouraged her to tell him what was wrong. Caroline confessed that she'd felt shut out of Art's life since the shooting. She pointed out that he spent all his free time with other officers and not with her. She could hear him talking on the telephone to them about things he hadn't told her. She was envious and jealous of his female squad members and began to worry that Art was attracted to one of them.

Art was shocked. Since the shooting, he felt Caroline had been his rock and anchor, that she kept him together by merely being there. He was compelled to be with others who had been at the scene and were police folks, and he admittedly felt more comfortable in the police station because he couldn't relax at home. But he regarded Caroline as the glue that kept him from falling apart. Once they had this discussion, Caroline felt less depressed and anxious, and Art became aware that he needed to make more of an effort to communicate both thoughts and feelings to Caroline.

After a trauma, intimates, friends, and family members are at risk for absorbing or catching each other's feelings. You may find yourself reliving your cop's incident in your head. You might obsess about what you were doing at the time and how grotesque it is that while your loved one was in jeopardy you were doing something else and didn't know. This is called vicarious traumatization, and it happens between people who love and care for each other.

Occasionally, a psychologically injured person will project some of his or her unbearable feelings onto you, and you may feel the same emotions that the injured person has experienced, such as helplessness, fear, abandonment, self-loathing, hopelessness, or depression. This can happen between people who are close simply because they *are* close.

For example, the more anxious and panicked Lilly felt after her shooting, the more anxious Jack became. He found himself giving her superficial advice. The harder he tried, the more irritated she seemed. He was growing more frustrated as she was becoming more impatient with his failed attempts to be supportive. Finally he realized he had "caught" her helplessness. He decided to put his cards on the table: He told her that he was feeling helpless to relieve her discomfort and guilty because he assumed it was his responsibility to fix it. They compared notes on their respective experiences of helplessness and wound up laughing at themselves. Weren't they a "poster couple"—the halt leading the lame?

Tips for Helping Yourself When Your Cop Is in Crisis

- Consider attending a family debriefing; for more information about the pros and cons of debriefings, see Chapter 6, page 116.
- Join a support group. Find out if family members are part of a department peer support team.
- If you need professional assistance, get it. Your mate may have benefits that include free, confidential visits for family members with an employee assistance program. Or your family may have medical insurance that includes psychiatric consultation. Seek out a counselor with some knowledge of police culture.
- Try not to bottle your feelings inside. If you have no one to talk to, write a letter or draw a picture about what you are experiencing emotionally. You don't have to mail the letter or show the picture to anyone else: It may just help you get your feelings out. Pay attention to the movies and dialogues that go on in your head. They are vital clues to what you are feeling. Pay attention to your dreams for the same reason.
- Recognize that you, too, may be suffering from the breakdown of adaptive denial. It was other people's mates who got hurt or became emotionally distressed—not yours. Yours was stronger, hardier, better trained, and so on. Allow yourself to have these feelings. It is normal to be disappointed when someone falls off the pedestal, even when you had put that person there in the first place.
- Establish reasonable goals for your "new normal." Back to the way it was is probably impossible. Reasonable priorities for recovery will be specific, measurable, and achievable. For instance, "I would like our family to be able to go on an outing together at least once a month" is a far more reasonable request than to want everything to be the way it was and for

(cont.)

(continued from previous page)

all of us to be happy again—which is an understandable wish but neither measurable nor realistic.

- Think about what would bring closure to the situation for you. Be prepared that this may not be the same for your loved one. For cops involved in a shooting, closure sometimes comes after the first anniversary, when the limit on civil liability is ended. For you, closure may come when the officer returns to work or has regained his or her sense of humor.
- Monitor your own self-talk. Your interpretation of a problem is crucial to your response. As an example, if your spouse is unaffectionate or disinterested in sex, it may be a mistake to assume that you are unlovable. Your cop may be unaffectionate because he or she has been traumatized and can't perform sexually. Challenge your negative assumptions. Communicate with your spouse.
- Don't try to make everything all right. In your wish to get back to normal, you may work too hard to make holidays happy and birthdays the way they were before. You may need to adjust to things the way they are, at least for a short time, rather than try to swim against the tide. If things don't change, you might decide to take more active steps.
- Listen to your body: If you have a lump in your throat, you may need to cry or to talk. Muscle tensions and gut aches might mean you are holding some anger inside. Depression may feel like a weight on your heart or your chest.

CHAPTER 8

KIDS AND TRAUMA

We had all wanted the simplest thing, to love and be
loved and be safe together, but we had lost it, and I
didn't know how to get it back.
—DOROTHY ALLISON, *Bastard Out of Carolina*

If families are at risk for "catching" trauma, children are the most
vulnerable family members because they are still learning how to
manage their emotions. Children and adolescents, however mature they appear, usually don't have the social or psychological
maturity to understand what has happened to them or to their
families when traumatic stress occurs.

Children respond to disruptions in the family according to
their age. Younger children will be more concerned with issues of
separation and safety: "Will Daddy be killed?" "Will I have to
live somewhere else?" Young children are particularly at risk because they do not have the language needed to put their feelings
into words, and as you now know, putting a traumatic experience
into words is how you resolve or soften the experience.

Older children are sensitive to being in the spotlight. If the
trauma that affected your family made the news, your children
may be exposed to unwanted attention from classmates, teachers,
and friends. They'll need help in preparing to face their friends,
and you'll need to ask them for brief updates about how things
are going. Help them work out some acceptable responses to the
attention they anticipate, and rehearse these responses in advance
so they don't have to think them up on the spot.

Adolescents are particularly sensitive to humiliation and to issues involving authority. They may be angry at Dad for exercising authority in his job and not at all sympathetic to his concerns or injuries. On the other hand, they may be frightened by the realization that Mom is not invulnerable to injury or stress and yet unable to talk to her about their fears because they seem childish. They may shrug off your attempts to talk with "I don't know" or "I don't care" or "Whatever."

PROVIDING A SAFE HAVEN

The family is a holding environment, a safe haven for children and adults to learn about managing the social and emotional aspects of life. A traumatic incident threatens the security of that environment.

Children are like litmus paper: They soak up tensions in their environment. When something bad happens to their parents or between their parents, they become emotionally upset in proportion to their parents' upset. It is no use telling them everything is okay when it isn't; that only sends the message that their own sense of reality is not to be trusted.

Children will respond to a critical incident, even if the incident was minor or happened to someone else. It's very common for kids whose parents have been only peripherally involved in a shooting to worry that their parents will get shot. They need to talk about their worries and be reassured. One officer, who was sick at home when a coworker was shot and killed, told me her oldest child called her at work every day for two weeks to see if she was okay. This child had never before been anxious about her mother's safety.

Restoring Normalcy

Because children are sensitive to their environment, do your best during a crisis to keep quarrels and disagreements to a minimum. Try to stick to a normal schedule for mealtimes and bedtimes. Let children know that they're still expected to do homework and household tasks. Feed them familiar foods, and try to let them sleep in their own beds.

As quickly as possible after a critical incident or other disruption, restore the protective umbrella of the family. Reassure children that while Mommy is upset and crying a lot, this is temporary. Tell them Daddy had a bad experience. Ask them if they ever felt sad or frightened by something. Find out what helped them. It will normalize things to relate the parent's upsetting experiences to something the child already knows or has experienced. For example, children may remember how sad they felt when a friend moved away or a pet died. They may recall being scared during a storm or when lost. Helping your children talk about what they or the family did to feel better will help them feel less helpless and more optimistic. They'll remember that eventually the sad parts went away and don't hurt so much anymore.

Giving Reassurance

During a crisis, try to give extra time to your children. This may be hard because you may have extra things to do yourself. Depending on the severity of the trauma or the upset to the family, you may need to have several talks with your kids. The point of your talks is to wean your child from continuous worry and restore a sense of security. Be reassuring, and be realistic. It is crucial that your child can depend on you to tell the truth.

Take five-year-old Gus, for instance. Gus's father, Jules, was bruised and shaken up after a frightening, brutal, humiliating fight in which he almost lost his gun. One day, shortly after the fight, Gus leaped into Jules's lap without warning. Jules, still highly adrenalized and easily startled, reflexively slapped Gus in the face. He then cried with shame and sorrow for hurting his son, who was being a normal, playful, affectionate kid. Jules, who hadn't told Gus what had happened, apologized profusely. He worked to restore his son's trust and to undo the message he had inadvertently sent—that violence toward another was the way to handle fear and anger. He started by telling his son, in child language, the story of what happened at work.

It was a very sad story. Jules hated losing that fight and particularly hated having to admit it to Gus. And, as much as he wanted to, he knew he couldn't promise Gus that he would never get beaten up again. But he did talk about how careful he would be. When Gus asked what would happen if Jules was shot, Jules reassured him that if he got hurt again and had to go to the hospital, Grandpa or Aunt Mary or friends next door would come right over and take Gus to their house until Mommy or Daddy came home. And Gus could take his toys along. This kind of reassurance is important to all children, especially to those with single parents. Jules didn't try to tell Gus this could never happen again or to persuade Gus to be a big boy and not cry. He realized how the incident that had disrupted his own life had brought uncertainty and fear into Gus's life too.

Understanding Emotions

Adolescents often hide their true feelings because they're trying to be independent. One of their worst fears is to be seen as abnormal, even when their reactions are totally normal. On occasion, teens will express their distress, not by clinging as young children do, but by acting out—taking chances, talking back, getting into trouble. They are like adults in this regard. They want to numb themselves or distract themselves from their own uncomfortable feelings. They may feel vengeful toward the person who hurt their parents, or they may feel—and this is likely in a public safety family—that they must step in and be the adult. Be on the alert and help them understand how their behavior is linked to whatever traumatic event has affected their family.

Frankie, age 14, was humiliated when his father got into a shoot-out with a drug dealer and it made all the headlines. He took a lot of razzing at school about his "Deadeye Dad" but never told his family. Although Frankie didn't experiment with drugs, some of his friends did, and they told him they weren't coming by his house anymore because his Dad would probably shoot them on the spot.

Instead of confronting his friends, he confronted his father: "Why did you have to shoot at the guy? Couldn't you have gassed him or shot him in the leg?" All were questions his classmates had taunted him with. When his Dad, who was understandably angry and hurt at Frankie's unsympathetic reaction, yelled at him for having lousy friends, Frankie stormed out of the house and didn't come home that night.

Frankie's Mom found out about the razzing at school when she called Frankie's homeroom teacher the next day to see if he was there. She asked the teacher to intervene on Frankie's behalf, and when he said he didn't have time, she had the distinct impression that the teacher didn't like cops and was subsequently unsympathetic to Frankie's problems.

Frankie's parents called a family meeting when Frankie came home. Everyone talked about how and what he or she had been feeling since the shooting. Dad said he was scared and worried about going back to work and hurt by Frankie's behavior. Mom said she was tired of keeping the peace between Frankie and his father and tired because she was doing everything at home. Frankie said he was angry at both his father and his friends because they each expected different things from him, and he was confused. No matter what he did, he didn't seem able to please anyone.

Frankie's family listened carefully. It was clear that Frankie thought he should be doing something to help his parents but didn't know what or how to make a difference. They gave him some concrete tasks he could do for his father and relieved him of the unrealistic expectations he shouldered as an only child. They also reassured him that his father was really okay but needed some time to get back on his feet emotionally. They sympathized with his pain at being ostracized by his friends and helped him to consider how he could deal with the razzing. They resisted the temptation to get angry at something or someone else: the shooter, Frankie's friends, the job, or each other. Instead they acknowledged that each of them was feeling the strain of what had happened, and they concentrated on working things out together.

Parents can help children manage their emotions by coaching them. Coaching children means that you help them think about their emotions and express them in acceptable ways. Someone smart once said, "You may not find something good in every experience, but there is always something to learn." Helping your child cope with a parent's trauma can be an opportunity for the child to mature and for you to become closer as a family.

Children from public safety families may be natural helpers or problem solvers just because they come from such a family.

Giving them something to do will focus their attention and help them feel confident, provided the task is suited to their abilities. A special chore will help them feel they're contributing to the family's well-being. Praise them for their help, and let them know how much it means.

It is important to set limits on unacceptable behavior while recognizing that there are no unacceptable feelings. It helps to separate behavior from feelings and feelings from self-esteem. Because I feel frightened doesn't mean I'm a coward. Or in Frankie's case, he was mad at his father, but that didn't mean he didn't love him as well. He needed to talk about his angry feelings, and his parents needed to hold him accountable for walking out of the house in anger. On the other hand, they had to help him challenge his own impulse control by acknowledging how hard it was for him to feel so angry and confused.

One way to normalize your children's feelings or to help them open up is to share your own feelings. Like Gus and Jules, it's wise to do this in a way that doesn't overwhelm or frighten your child. This may be contrary to the common wisdom that parents must remain strong and certain at all times.

I watched the children of a recently widowed woman scramble to comfort their mother who was sobbing in a public place. They rallied around her, trying to comfort her and pleading with her to stop crying—a difficult task for two small children who were themselves still reeling from their father's death only months earlier. Later on, after adult friends helped the mother regain emotional control, I found myself sitting with the children, who were staring off into space with that 1,000-mile stare we have come to associate with intense stress.

Because I didn't know them well, I wasn't sure what to say, although I wanted to acknowledge their feelings. I said that when my father became ill and died, I, too, felt helpless to console or guide my mother through those troubled times even though I was a grownup. I told them that she eventually got through it on her own and that the best I could do was listen to her troubles. They looked at me with amazement. I had essentially told them that it was normal to feel helpless under some circumstances, that even adults feel helpless at times, and that some things will go away on their own. It wasn't much, but it seemed to help.

Giving Information

Like adults, children need information to quell their anxiety. They may ask the same questions over and over. Give your children enough information to help them understand what has happened and only as much as they can tolerate without becoming confused or upset. Think about what kind of information they might want and at what level of detail.

It's not advisable to provide younger children with dramatic stories or graphic details that may frighten them. Young children often have a distorted or magical understanding of things. Check their understanding by asking them to repeat what they heard, or let them tell you the story of what happened. Older children may want and need more detail, and they may be interested in media reports of the event. All children need guidance with the media. For example, the ongoing barrage of replays of airplanes crashing into the World Trade Center, the Pentagon, and the field in Pennsylvania gave some children the impression that hundreds of planes were crashing all over the United States. A national survey after 9/11 found that children exposed to the catastrophe solely through television experienced symptoms of stress-related trauma, some for as long as two years. The level of stress was associated with the extent of their TV viewing.

The day after Mickey's dad was shot and killed in the line of duty, the television was filled with reports that misrepresented his father's actions. The suspect's family and their lawyer claimed police brutality. Mickey's uncle and some of his father's friends talked to Mickey about these claims, provided him with accurate information, and listened to his concerns. His TV viewing needed to be monitored. Ultimately, his uncle, who was also a law enforcement officer, gave a TV interview of his own to balance the publicity that seemed engineered to prepare a defense for the suspect's indefensible actions. Mickey's entire family was outraged by the media.

Dealing with Delayed Reactions

Children from the same family will have unique reactions to crisis and, like adults, are subject to delayed traumatic responses. Sgt. Gary Sommers, testifying before the House Select Committee on

Children, Youth, and Families during the 102nd Congress, told a poignant story about accidentally killing his best friend and colleague, Mark, on a SWAT team raid. His three young children reacted differently to this tragedy. His seven-year-old was angry because his parents were away a lot, and their normal family routine was disrupted. His five-year-old was furious that Gary had killed Mark, who was a friend to the whole family. And his daughter, who was three at the time of the shooting, turned to her father two years later as he was putting her to bed and asked, "Daddy, why did you kill Mark?" Remember that children do not have any real sense of death or injury as a permanent state until the age of six or seven.

Don't be surprised by a delayed reaction, and don't overlook the possibility that today's puzzling behavior may relate to something that happened much earlier in your child's world. Talking to each other can help you and your child make sense of the connection between past and present.

Dealing with Separations

One of the unique issues affecting law enforcement families is the fact that in the face of a natural disaster, such as a flood or earthquake, officers must go to work. During Hurricane Katrina, 85% of the local officers lost their homes. Some decided to leave their posts and look after their families. Others did not. It was an agonizing time for everyone. With all communication systems wiped out or spotty at best, the emergency responders didn't know if their families and homes were safe, and families didn't know if their loved ones were in danger.

Lucinda was called into work after a serious earthquake. She had to tear herself away from her two small children, who were utterly terrified by the shaking and crashing all around them. Her husband stayed with the kids, but he was angry to be left alone with the cleanup and the prospect of aftershocks. He felt it was too much to do to cope with the kids' distress and deal with the mess in the house. He wanted Lucinda to stay while he checked for structural damage and reassured himself that their house was safe to inhabit.

Lucinda felt torn in two. She had to go into work. There was a threat of looting, traffic was chaotic, and the number of trapped and injured people was still undetermined, but it was likely to be high. Her kids were screaming for their mommy, and her sergeant was screaming for her.

She promised to call home as often as possible. When she did, her husband was irritable and frustrated, and the kids were miserable. Lucinda was the primary homemaker, and Jeff knew very little about their daily habits. Because of the stress, the children were clingy and demanding. They sought comfort in familiar routines and familiar foods. Her husband paged Lucinda constantly to ask questions and got furious when she couldn't return his page immediately. She, on the other hand, was angry at his lack of empathy for her dilemma. It was an overwhelming experience for everyone, and it took weeks for the family to stop feeling hurt and angry. To add insult to injury, Lucinda felt taken advantage of at work as she spent a lot of time waiting around while her commander developed an incident response plan.

In the best of all possible worlds, families should prepare disaster plans, including plans for communicating with each other, perhaps through a third party (such as grandparents) located in a different region; local calls in a disaster area are often blocked by an "all circuits are busy" message immediately after a catastrophe, but a call to an outside area code can have a better chance of getting through. Make contingency plans for locating the kids if they are at school or elsewhere during a disaster, and plan a backup place to reunite as a family, such as a community center, in case your home is in an area that is evacuated or unreachable.

Afterward, everyone will need to talk about how he or she felt and what happened to them when they all were separated. Small kids may need to draw pictures or act out their experiences with hand puppets or toys. Sometimes it helps to let your child dictate his or her own story to you while you write it down in a blank book. Your child can add pictures and then look at the book whenever he or she wants to. Be sure to include whatever positive memories your child has along with the scary ones.

SIGNS AND SYMPTOMS: HOW KIDS RESPOND TO TRAUMA

The following signs and symptoms are typical of the way children respond to trauma. They are normal reactions, but if they persist unabated after two to six weeks, you might consider getting professional consultation.

Temper Tantrums

Anger, hostility, tantrums, mood swings, and other unruly behavior may be an expression of your child's fear or helplessness. Try to uncover what is going on rather than react. This, of course, is easier said than done, especially if your child throws a tantrum as you are rushing out the door to work, the phone is ringing, and the dog has run into the street.

Try to help your child find other ways to express feelings besides tantrums. Encourage him or her to use toys to relieve tension such as hand puppets, finger paints, soft toys, or pillows they can hit. Older children may be able to talk it out or write stories, poems, or journals about what is bothering them. They can write letters they never mail or write pretend newspaper stories. Listen to what your children say as they play. You can learn a lot about what is bothering them and then use their own language to communicate.

Help children accept their feelings as normal reactions to an abnormal event—the disruption in their parents' lives and their own lives. Help them find ways to ask for what they want and need. If the afflicted parent is too preoccupied to pay attention to them, help them find ways to ask for something they may reasonably expect. For example, Dave and his son, Todd, were used to going to basketball games until Dave became too uncomfortable in large, unruly crowds. It softened Todd's disappointment when his father agreed instead to watch a game on television in the security of their home and throw hoops together at a local ball court.

Aches and Pains

Because young children are often not able to use words for their feelings, they may turn their feelings into a variety of physical ailments—stomach aches, headaches, and so on—for which there is no medical cause. Sometimes this is part of a ruse to stay home because they are too anxious to be separated from Mom or Dad.

It's important, again, to get them to talk, to reassure them that they will be okay, to acknowledge that things are tough on them, and then to firmly but gently insist that they continue their normal routines and responsibilities.

Guilt and Responsibility

Kids have an uncanny way of assuming responsibility for things over which they have no control. Children of divorce often have to be repeatedly reassured that the divorce did not occur because of anything they did or didn't do. Lani's children were certain they were responsible for her car crash because they "forgot" to ask her guardian angel to look out for her that day. Lani had to reassure them that the bad guys she was chasing caused the crash and that the guardian angels helped her from being more seriously hurt.

Bedtime Troubles

When children are upset or anxious, they often have trouble sleeping or going to bed. This is a common occurrence and an upsetting one since sleep deprivation makes things worse, and bedtime may be the only time you and your mate have for yourselves. The following guidelines may help.

- It is okay to delay bedtime when a child is anxious and wants to talk. But set a limit first. Use a timer.
- When your children are afraid to sleep alone, try spending some extra time in their bedrooms, reassuring them. If that's not enough, allow the children to sleep in your bedroom on a mattress on the floor or in a sibling's room. Ideally this arrangement should not last longer than three to four days, and this limit should be established in advance. Be firm in your commitment to return to normal sleeping arrangements within that time period.
- Make sure you're not inadvertently communicating fears of your own or that you need the child's company in your bedroom as much as he or she needs yours.
- Get your child a nightlight. Leave the door ajar. Leave the

closet light on. Get a big stuffed animal for your child to sleep with.

• Make sure you're spending enough time with your child during the day.

• If your children come out of their rooms, return them calmly and reassure them you're nearby. Getting angry, punishing, spanking, or shouting rarely helps.

• If your children have nightmares, try these techniques: Encourage them to draw the nightmare in a storybook. Talk with your children about how they can fight back in their dreams. Draw a picture of them yelling at the bad person who hurt their parent. Encourage them to yell at nightmare monsters, telling the monsters to go away and get out of their dreams.

School Phobias and Problems

Some children will be so fearful of being separated from a parent that they'll refuse to go to school. It is important to be firm and let your children know you expect them to attend. School phobias, if they become entrenched, can be hard to reverse, so you should stand firm on this. Do, however, find out from your children what is so upsetting. Are they afraid to let Mom or Dad out of their sight? Are they being teased? Are people talking about their parents?

Talk to your children's teachers and tell them what happened. Teachers need to know that your children are under some stress and may be distracted, have difficulty concentrating, want to go home, or be unable, at least temporarily, to complete class assignments on time. Advise the teachers what to tell other students, if anything. Teachers need accurate information so they can stop rumors. The information they give to the other students should be simple and not overwhelming. Teachers can help the other students know what or what not to say to your kids. Alert school counselors; find a safe haven in school in the form of a responsible, empathic adult to whom your children can turn if they are getting teased or taunted.

When children are distressed or worried, they have trouble concentrating, which can show up at homework time. Acknowledge that this may be the case, and make some reasonable allowances with the understanding that you expect the usual homework habits to be back in force in a few days.

Your children may need more help with homework than usual. Help out if you are able to do so. If not, solicit help from a friend, neighbor, or family member. Set a reasonable time limit for studying, taking the extra issues into account. Or, break up studying time into smaller segments. Your children may be able to concentrate for 15 minutes at a time but not 30. Increase the study time to accommodate your children's abilities, and reward their progress.

Use breaks and time-out periods to defuse tension and anxiety. Give children a timer, and let them set it themselves.

Keep your expectations reasonable. If your children are truly distressed, their ability to perform will decrease. Accept "good enough" schoolwork for the time being.

Phobias and Avoidant Behavior

On occasion, children will develop phobias or avoidant behavior. After the Loma Prieta and Northridge earthquakes in California, many children (and adults) were afraid to be inside. Time and a lot of authentic reassurance help. It is never a good idea to give false reassurance, such as "We will never have another earthquake," because when the next one occurs, your children will think you lied to them and that you can't be counted on.

Regressive Behavior

Regressive behavior—children acting younger than they are—is a typical response to stress, and you may expect to see your young children wetting the bed or trying to crawl into yours. They may be more needy or clingy than usual. They may demand to be held or fed. They may whine, cry, and suck their thumbs. Older children, who are comfortable doing things for themselves, may suddenly want Mom or Dad to help them or to do the things for them. This is a temporary stress reaction and will most likely pass in a few days.

These "childish" behaviors should never be ridiculed. Children respond to praise. Make an effort to reward and acknowledge your child's mature behavior rather than focusing on the immature.

WHEN TO GET PROFESSIONAL HELP

If the behavioral changes you note in your children do not pass or diminish in intensity or frequency in two to six weeks, consider consulting your pediatrician, your rabbi or minister, the department psychologist, or some other helping professional who understands children, adolescents, traumatic response, and the police culture.

Consider consulting a professional if your child becomes excessively *hypervigilant* or *fearful* or engages in *repetitive play* about the incident. Children use repetition to get a sense of mastery. Almost all children have a favorite storybook they want to hear over and over until they can recite it word for word. By contrast, repetitive play is more like a broken record when the needle is stuck in the same groove. It is as though your child cannot move forward.

Behaviors that seriously impede your child's normal routine or serious acting out should at least prompt you to seek telephone consultation. Any radical change in mood, behavior, or basic eating or sleeping habits that lasts more than a few weeks should also signal the need for professional consultation. The same would be true if your children are emotionally constricted, listless, socially withdrawn, or disinterested in their usual activities. Acting out aggressively, major loss of appetite accompanied by weight loss, and suicidal or homicidal thoughts or threats require immediate professional attention.

Trauma can strike a family that is already under stress or one in which the marriage is already strained. If your family was under stress prior to the trauma, you may want to consider contacting a helping professional before you see any signs and symptoms in your children or yourself. You may be relieved to have a neutral third party available to help, to give feedback or to address those underlying tensions that may now be made worse by the recent crisis. Read Chapter 11, about getting help when you need it, for more information.

Tips for Helping Children Deal with Their Parents' Crisis

- Explore rather than ignore what your child is feeling by listening carefully. Accept that you won't and don't need to have all the answers. Don't get anxious about this, and don't try to solve your child's problem before you understand it.
- Explore alternate ways of dealing with feelings. Encourage your child to come up with ideas so that your child learns how to problem-solve.
- Reassure your children that anger, sadness, fear, and other feelings are normal under the circumstance.
- Try to stay on an even keel. Your children are likely to imitate the way the adults they know cope with trauma and will react more to their parents' emotional responses than to the event itself.

EMOTIONAL EXTREMES

CHAPTER 9

DOMESTIC ABUSE
The Best-Kept Secret Shame of Policing

> Police officers are required by law to effect an arrest
> in cases of domestic violence in which there is
> evidence to support the abuse. The law does not
> make exceptions for circumstances in which the
> abuser is a police officer.
> —LT. JOHN FELTGEN, *Police Chief*

Domestic violence in police families occurs more than we think and is rarely talked about, until it makes headlines.

- April 26—A police chief shoots his wife and kills himself in front of their children.
- June 28—A four-year veteran was suspended and stripped of his gun and badge for beating up his girlfriend.
- July 7—A rookie and a 12-year veteran were each accused of assaulting their girlfriends. One officer was arrested, the other put on modified duty.
- July 10—Two veteran officers were put on light duty for threatening their respective mates with guns.
- August 15—A veteran cop killed her boyfriend after he beat her badly.
- August 24—A cop was placed on modified duty, and his gun taken away, after he became a suspect in the murder of his pregnant girlfriend.

BEHIND THE HEADLINES: JENNY'S STORY

Jenny's counselor gave me her journal. Writing a journal was the way Jenny went about healing from years of physical and emotional abuse. She gave her counselor permission to show others the journal because she hoped to break the silence and help others the way she had been helped.

"Actually, it was because he was a cop that I didn't call anyone. I knew they'd cover up for him like they did for each other. Just look the other way. Or maybe some of the guys he supervised would use this to get at him, and he'd lose his job and blame it on me. I didn't want him arrested or fired, I just wanted him to stop hurting me.

"It didn't start right away. At first it was so intermittent I thought he was just having a bad day, no big deal. Mostly it was verbal. Sometimes he threw things, plates of food, cups of coffee, the remote control. He didn't hit me, but he meant to.

"One day he threw a full can of soda at me because I was five minutes late getting off from work. It hit me on the head, and I needed stitches. At the hospital he told them I fell. When they wanted to take X-rays, he made me refuse because he didn't want me to be where he couldn't hear what I said.

"Another time I was talking on the telephone with my sister, and he got upset and started choking me. I wanted to believe he just lost his temper and wasn't going to do it again. He hated when I got together with my family. He made things so unpleasant I saw less and less of them.

"The abuse got worse after I got pregnant for the first time. We were remodeling our kitchen, and he was upset because I couldn't help with the heavy stuff anymore. He made me do it anyway, and I miscarried in my sixth month. Later he blamed me for losing the baby.

"He always apologized and promised never to hurt me again. I wanted him to change, and I thought I had to believe in him so he would. I told myself, 'He isn't beating me, he's just hitting.' I know that sounds crazy, but at the time I thought there was a difference. After all, I didn't end up like you see on television with broken bones. I never needed surgery. He would tell me it was okay because he hit me with an open hand and didn't punch me. When the punching started later on, it wasn't where anybody would see it. He would hit me on the leg, in the ribs, on my back, or in my stomach.

"After I had my first child, he got frustrated because I couldn't give him undivided attention. He would sit in front of the TV set and say, 'Get me something to eat,' and I would. I was still working and had to ask his permission to do anything other than my normal go-to-work-and-come-home routine. I even had to ask permission to go to the supermarket.

"Looking back, I see he must have felt he lost control over me when I first started working. From that day on, I had to tell him what I did every minute of the day. After a while he even started driving me to and from work.

"For years he threatened that if I tried to leave him he would kill me or take the kids and never let me see them again. I believed he was capable of doing both. Sometimes he'd clean his gun while we argued. He threatened to shoot me and get rid of my body. He told me he knew how to do this. He said he would chop my body up and put it through a wood chipper. He would go into detail. I was always afraid, but I was most afraid of him taking the kids. I was stressed to the max. I felt like such a bad mother, and I thought no one would believe in me.

"I could see how this was affecting my children. My son started imitating his father and smart-mouthing me. Later he told me he was mad at me for not keeping his father happy so he wouldn't get angry, hit me, and yell at the kids. My daughter, on the other hand, was furious with her father. She tried to intervene when he got physical and told me, 'If Daddy hurts you again, I'm gonna hurt him.' She was only 11. I was terrified he would begin hitting her too.

"Once we were sitting in the car, and he hit me. Somebody saw this, took down our license plate, and called the police. Of course the plate came back registered to him. He knew the cops who showed up at the house and told them it was a mistake, that whoever called misread the plate. I was in the bathroom with a bloody nose, but he told them I went out. He knew they wouldn't come in because they didn't have a warrant. So they just stood around shooting the breeze. Anyhow, I knew no one would believe he hit me because he's the kind of guy who's always stopping to help someone, and he has the letters of commendation to prove it. I had so many bruises on my face I couldn't go to work the next day.

"I think the thing that bothered me most was the lies. I had to lie to my family and to my friends and to my boss whenever they asked me what was wrong or how I got hurt. The month before I left him, it was an everyday thing. He was hitting me in the arms and face where the bruises were visible. I felt stupid. I was a grown-up and knew I had to deal with my problems, but I didn't know how. I didn't feel like anyone could protect me, especially if we were still living together. Staying safe monopolized my life. All I could think about was how to keep him calm. I was constantly walking on eggshells.

"Finally, I called a domestic abuse hotline and talked to a counselor. I told her, 'I don't want to make this sound worse than it is.' She said, 'Don't you realize it *is* worse than you're making it out to be?' "

AN OVERVIEW OF THE FACTS

According to the U.S. Department of Justice's findings on intimate partner violence (IPV), the number of nonfatal violent crimes committed against women in the United States has declined by nearly half since 1993, and the number of fatal crimes by 22%. But reader beware: Despite vigorous law enforcement efforts and changes in the law, domestic abuse remains a major problem, one that is greatly underreported and therefore almost certainly underestimated.

• In 2001, approximately 588,490 intimate partner crimes were committed against women and 103,220 against men. That means that 85% of all battering victims were women, and 20% of all nonfatal violent crimes against women were committed by someone they knew.
• In 2000, 1,247 women and 440 men were killed by an intimate partner.
• On average, three American women are murdered by their husbands or boyfriends every day. That makes a woman's chances of being murdered by her partner greater than that of a police officer being murdered on the job.

• Between 1998 and 2002, 49% of 3.5 million reported and unreported instances of family violence were crimes against spouses. The most frequent type of crime was simple assault. About three-fourths of the partner victims were female, and three-fourths of the partner perpetrators were male.

• Twenty to 30% of married couples experience domestic violence at some point during their relationship.

• Ninety-one percent of all attacks on women are precipitated by their attempts to leave an abusive relationship. Disintegrating families are highly at risk, and women who leave abusive partners remain at risk.

• Domestic violence is a leading cause of injuries to women ages 15 to 44.

• Twice the number of women are raped by their husbands or ex-husbands than are raped by strangers.

• Men who batter women also batter their children. Children of abused mothers are 57 times more likely to be harmed by IPV between their parents than children of nonabused mothers.

• Between 4 and 8% of pregnant women are abused at least once during their pregnancy.

• The battering of pregnant women causes more birth defects than the diseases for which children are usually immunized.

• Each year, between 3 and 10 million American children are at risk for witnessing domestic violence in their homes.

• Alcohol and drug abuse do not cause domestic violence but may be associated with it. Batterers who drink or use drugs have two separate problems that need to be treated independently.

COPS WHO BATTER

If you are reading this because you or someone you know is being abused, your first obligation is safety. Turn immediately to page 178, the section titled "Staying Safe," and to the tips that follow. If you are unclear about whether a relationship is abusive, turn to page 170, the section titled "Are You Being Abused?"

The frequency or prevalence of domestic abuse among police families is difficult to pin down as so little research has been done on the subject. Getting at the truth is hard because officers and their spouses are unlikely to voluntarily admit, even in a confidential survey, to committing an illegal act that might get them fired. Still, *if* domestic violence occurs in police families at the same rate it does in the general population, then about 60,000 to 180,000 police households could be affected. On the other hand, some people argue that it occurs less in law enforcement families because preemployment screening, background checks, and polygraphs weed out most of the actual or potential abusers.

In 1996, the Behavioral Science Unit of the FBI sponsored a week-long conference on domestic abuse in police families. There were 34 papers presented by police professionals, psychologists, and academics. I recently read the conference proceedings that were published in 2000. There was little agreement among the authors about a number of issues: how widespread the problem is, what causes cops to be abusive—abuse suffered in their own childhoods, personality problems, changes resulting from their work, and so on—what kind of preemployment screening adequately identifies abusers, what to do about abusive officers, and how and when to do it. The only point of agreement was a zero-tolerance policy for bona fide incidents of abuse. If professionals are still arguing about how big or bad this problem is, how can police families make sense of it?

When I began updating this chapter, I heard from a colleague who was quite concerned that estimates of police family abuse had been blown way out of proportion. What message do we send to an abusive officer, he wondered, if we say that this behavior is so commonplace that it is the norm? He sent me some statistics from a "small" sample of 12,000 police applicants in which 7% of all applicants admitted to striking a romantic partner. Since only half of the entire group was hired, he found it unlikely that a known abuser would be among them. Another colleague, using a similar screening device, reported that 10% of 1,458 applicants admitted to hitting a romantic partner. He followed up on this group and found that only one of the admitted batterers became a police officer.

Do these examples and others too numerous to include mean that preemployment screening works to keep abusers out of law enforcement? Evidence indicates it is helping, *if*—and that's a big *if*—it is properly administered in coordination with a thorough background check and a polygraph. Polygraphs are especially important screening tools because they greatly increase the percentage of applicants willing to admit to problems and illegal behavior.

WHAT PUTS COPS AT RISK TO BECOME ABUSERS?

A colleague who has devoted decades of her professional life to the study of domestic violence told me she believes cops are the most dangerous of all abusers and their spouses are the most endangered. She says this because cops have guns and will use them; they are accustomed to using verbal and physical force or the threat of it to get citizens to do what they want; and they know how the legal system works and where the battered women's shelters are.

All the hazardous habits described in Chapter 2 place officers at risk for domestic violence: emotional control, cynicism and overprotectiveness, being chained to the chain of command, and hypervigilance. Cops want to be in control. They have high expectations for compliance and respect. They work in paramilitary organizations, where they both give and take orders without an explanation. Refusal to comply is considered insubordination as opposed to a difference of opinion. When citizens fail to comply, cops experience this as disrespectful and as a potential prelude to danger. It is their number one task to regain control of the situation.

Cops regard physical force and verbal intimidation as tools to get the job done. They may be desensitized to verbal, emotional, and physical violence because these are routine parts of their everyday work life. You, on the other hand, are not.

Two police psychologists from the Los Angeles County Sheriffs office, Audrey Honig and Elizabeth White, noted that for cops, restraining someone probably rates a two on a use-of-force scale that ranges from 1 to 10. Grabbing, shoving, and pushing also rank low. Punching, grappling, or using a restraint hold might equal a 5 or 6. A 10 would be reserved for drawing and shooting a gun. Raising their voices and using intimidating nonverbal tactics associated with a command presence wouldn't even rate a one.

But for the family, yelling might feel like a four, and grabbing or pushing might rate a six or seven. The other day, I asked a cop to help me reach something on top of a cabinet. As I pointed at what I wanted, he moved me out of the way so roughly I felt as though I'd been shoved. Later, I wondered if he was angry with me for asking him to help.

Although it is slowly changing, policing is still a man's world filled with macho values. "Real men" are often taught to ignore their feelings and are made to feel weak if they ask for help. They value action over talking things out, and anything that threatens their authority threatens their self-esteem. They may be more inclined to try to work things out with coworkers than with family members. They value traditional male and female roles—many of them grew up in homes where women were subservient and perhaps subjected to abuse—and fear losing face with their peers if they can't keep their mates and their kids in line. When this does happen, it becomes time to apply some control, or as one cop casually described wife beating to me, time to "tune up the old lady."

Our culture says a man's home is his castle. Some officers, particularly those with low self-worth and high levels of job dissatisfaction, seek to rectify their professional problems by asserting their authority at home. Their efforts to control the family serve to soothe themselves and reestablish their self-esteem. They depend too much on their jobs and their families as a source of self-worth. They can't seem to tolerate ordinary disagreements or differences of opinion that arise in any relationship. The possible loss of a job or a relationship is extremely threatening to their sense of well-being.

Although women are most often the victims of domestic abuse, they are not immune from being abusers. Women police applicants are more likely than males to admit to having slapped, punched, or injured a partner. A study published in 2000 took a sample of 857 Baltimore police officers. Nine percent of the respondents reported committing spousal abuse, and women officers were nearly twice as likely as males to report such behavior. In one of the studies I quoted in the first edition, police family violence was described as "mutual": Both husband and wife were physically abusive, although wives were much more likely to be physically injured and psychologically distressed as a result of violence. This raises a number of unanswered questions: Are women more scrupulously honest or confessional by nature? Are those who are attracted to policing more aggressive than their male counterparts? While screeners and researchers now make a sharper distinction between physical and verbal abuse, it remains unclear which acts of violence are offensive or defensive. This is an important point. Women may be more likely to act aggressively to protect themselves or their children, whereas men may act aggressively to wield power over their partners.

Here are other factors to consider:

- Ethnicity may be related to abusive behavior. The Baltimore study found that officers charged with domestic abuse were apt to be African American or Hispanic. And my colleague with the huge applicant database says that African Americans, Hispanics, and female applicants report having struck an intimate partner at twice the rate reported by white or Asian applicants. This holds true when facing a polygraph and before the Omnibus Appropriations Act (see below).
- Work conditions also come into play. In Baltimore, researchers concluded that officers who reported high levels of job stress were three times more likely to abuse their intimate partners. This echoes the conclusions of studies I quoted in 1997 that associated marital aggression with a number of work-related factors.
- Work assignment: Uniform patrol officers and narcotics officers had higher rates of domestic violence than those in other assignments. Narcotics officers were four times more likely to be physically violent at home than were officers working elsewhere.
- Working the midnight or swing shift.
- Working long hours—more than 50 hours per week—or taking no leave time.
- Sleep deprivation.
- Poor coping strategies such as "rugged individualism" or going it alone.
- Burnout and job dissatisfaction.
- Using more than 19 days of sick leave.

The suggestion that work stress contributes to domestic abuse is supported by several studies that found little evidence of domestic abuse among small rural or suburban agencies, the implication being that work stress is higher in large, high-crime, urban departments. On the other hand, the online study of police families that Dr. Lorraine Greene and I conducted suggested that larger departments offer more work options and have more available resources to help troubled officers and their families. Whether or not officers and their families make use of these resources is another question. Being able to ask for help from friends, family, peer supporters, or professionals can reduce isolation and the sensation of being out of control. Getting help just might head off some forms of domestic abuse. Unfortunately, many cops, male and female, are hesitant to ask because it will make them look or feel weak. And since many cops are reluctant to socialize outside of their profession, they tend to reinforce each other. More important, their families are often very isolated. Isolation is an important component of domestic abuse.

AMALIA'S STORY

Amalia and Hector met when he was a deputy sheriff and she was working as a communications dispatcher. They married a year later. At first they had a lot in common because they worked similar hours and shared similar stresses. Then Amalia's mother became ill, and Amalia left work to care for her. Hector resented her absence and her preoccupation. He was unable to console her when her mother eventually died.

Budget cuts and lack of seniority sent Hector back to corrections, where he felt like a second-class cop. Amalia got pregnant and gained a lot of weight. Hector started referring to her as a "fat pig" and monitored what and when she ate. He felt personally humiliated by her weight gain. At parties, he compared her to younger, thinner women and told her how bad she looked.

They decided she should be a stay-at-home mother, and after their first baby, Amalia started a home-based medical transcription business. Hector was still working the jail, feeling more and more frustrated. He hated his job, and he felt stuck; yet he supposedly couldn't make a change because he was burdened by the responsibility of a new child.

Amalia's transcription business, on the other hand, was doing well. There was ample money coming in, and she encouraged Hector to quit and find something more to his liking. But he was too fearful and lacked sufficient confidence to compete with others. He began to displace his frustration at home. He would go over Amalia's books and want her to account for every penny. He interrogated her about her clients and listened to her phone calls.

Amalia made an appointment with a marriage counselor, and Hector went along. He didn't like the counselor, and every time they went, he seemed to get angrier at Amalia. One night after a session, Hector grabbed Amalia by the arm hard enough to leave marks. He shook her and grabbed her around the throat. She called the local police and had him arrested that night for domestic battery. His department sent a special supervisory unit to the house, and they took photos to document Amalia's bruises.

Hector was booked and then released to go home and pack his bags. The police provided protective custody for Amalia and her child while this was happening.

Back at work, Hector was placed on administrative probation, sent for a psychological evaluation, and mandated to enroll in an anger control program. His weapon was taken away, and he was placed on modified duty. Because they live in a small town, the county prosecutor was asked to conduct the investigation in order to avoid any conflict of interest or any impression that the department was covering up for one of its own.

Hector complained that he was being made an example of because he was a cop. Amalia worried that if he was fired, they'd lose all their medical benefits. They saw separate counselors, although Amalia thought that Hector went only because he was ordered to and that he still didn't think what he had done was so bad. Ultimately, they filed for divorce.

Amalia has no regrets over having had Hector arrested. She is confident that she took the right steps to get the kind of support she needed to guarantee her continued safety. Only in an atmosphere of safety could she and Hector have tried to work on their problems. It would be hard to call Amalia's experience a success story, but it does illustrate what you can do in a bad situation. In contrast to Jenny, Amalia didn't endure years of abuse before asking for help. She drew the line at physical violence. Fortunately, Hector's department provided help and took appropriate action to punish him. These actions sent Hector (and his coworkers) a strong message that domestic violence would not be tolerated.

Amalia continues to get counseling. She has a supportive place to work on rebuilding her self-esteem, understanding her own personal history, and planning for her future. Starting her own business has really paid off because she and her child aren't entirely dependent on Hector for financial support.

ARE YOU BEING ABUSED?

This may strike you as a silly question: Wouldn't someone who is being abused know it? Not always. Couples can be in denial about relationship abuse. Jenny minimized her husband's violent behavior, perhaps as a strategy to keep herself safe or to feel less helpless and frightened than she actually was. She told herself, "He was just angry and lost his temper; he didn't punch me; I wasn't as bad off as people I see on television; I had no broken bones."

Her husband also justified the damage he did by blaming it on Jenny. He wouldn't have been so angry that he "had" to hit her if she had been on time. He also said open-hand hitting was not as bad as punching with a closed fist—although he eventually did that too. He softened his violent behavior with remorse and efforts to make it up to her, but over the years, his periods of regret and kindness grew shorter while the periods of violence became longer and more frequent.

Make no mistake about this: *Domestic abuse is not about anger.* All couples get angry and have fights. Partner abuse occurs when one partner uses anger or force to intimidate the other and to control his or her behavior. Ask yourself this: Am I afraid of my mate? Is my mate afraid of me? If you answer yes, you should seek help.

There's a lot of controversy among experts about domestic abuse: Is it one-sided or mutual? Does it reflect pathology or patriarchy? Although I'm not an expert in the field, it appears to me that there may be several types of domestic abuse. Dr. Susan Hanks, domestic violence expert, describes these variations as follows.

Stress-Related Abuse

Violence erupts in response to a crisis or unrelenting pressure, perhaps following a developmental milestone like the birth of a baby, acute illness, death of a family member, job loss, and so on. It is a rare occurrence, and both partners are horrified and alarmed by it. There is no history of other abuse, and the current incident is taken seriously and not discounted. The couple does not trivialize it with vague verbal descriptions such as "He went ballistic," when he kicked her so hard he left marks; or "Things just got out of hand," when he slapped her, pulled her hair, and threatened to kill her.

Each partner recognizes that this one act of violence has altered the balance of power in their relationship and instilled a sense of fear and threat. They acknowledge the negative impact on children who may have witnessed the abuse. Such a couple may respond well to individual, couple, or family therapy, and the abuser may ultimately learn to control his or her behavior.

For example, in Chapter 8, you read about Jules, who slapped his son, Gus, in the face when Gus startled him by jumping on him without warning. Jules had never hit Gus before and has not hit him since. He was remorseful for his actions, took responsibility for what happened, and then worked in therapy to repair his relationship with Gus and to recover from undiagnosed posttraumatic stress. Contrast Jules with Jenny's husband, who berated Jenny and their kids endlessly, yelling at them for the smallest mistakes or for not being able to read his mind and anticipate his needs.

Control-Related Abuse

The abuse is chronic and takes many forms. The abuser takes little or no responsibility for the abuse, blaming it all on the victim. He or she uses intimidation and violence to coerce and control others and to calm down. Obedience soothes the abuser's stormy psychological state.

Controlling abusers are excessively needy. Common troubles—a difference of opinion, a tired and unresponsive spouse, a failed promotion—can provoke them into a rage. These abusers have little sympathy for their victims. Their victims feel and act like hostages in their own homes and may have all the symptoms of PTSD, described in Chapter 5.

This kind of couple requires a lot of help, although couple or family therapy may be harmful until the violence has stopped and the abuser has taken responsibility for his or her actions. Couple therapy, especially with a counselor who is unfamiliar with the recognition and treatment of domestic violence, can agitate the situation and place the victim in harm's way. Even when violence is stopped, other forms of control and intimidation may persist or escalate.

Individual therapy or same-sex group therapy is most useful for this couple. The victim will need help recovering from physical and psychological damage. She may need practical assistance in locating medical care, safe housing, financial assistance, and legal consultation. Children may need therapy to deal with what they have seen, heard, or experienced. The abuser may respond to a structured, educational approach aimed at modifying harmful thought patterns and changing behavior.

Special Circumstances

There is some indication that soldiers and officers like Jules, who suffer from PTSD, may have an increased penchant for violent behavior. Although this may explain their actions, it does not absolve them of responsibility. The same is true for family violence that is associated with severe mental disorders and drug or alcohol addiction. Regardless of the cause of the problem, *it is the abusers' responsibility to control their own behavior and the victims' burden to keep themselves and their children safe.*

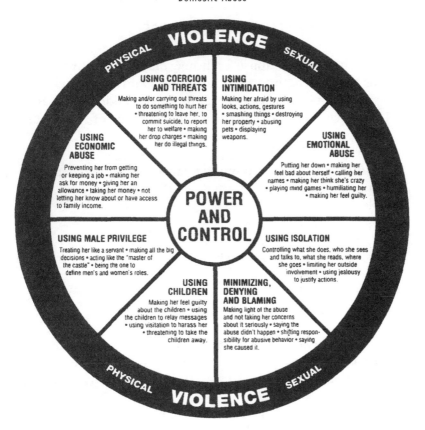

Power and Control Wheel. From Pence and Paymar (1993). Copyright 1993 by Springer Publishing Company, Inc., New York, NY 10012. Reprinted by permission.

If you have questions about what conduct is considered abusive, study the Power and Control Wheel (above), developed by the Duluth Domestic Abuse Intervention Project. This wheel gives you a complete picture of the wide range of abusive and coercive behaviors. I like it because it doesn't focus exclusively on violence, which is only the tip of the iceberg. The abusive and controlling behaviors described within the spokes of the wheel may persist for a long time before actual violence erupts. If you recognize any of these behaviors in your family, you need to attend to them quickly and with caution.

FAMILY ABUSE AND KIDS

Children who witness abuse at home may suffer psychological problems that extend into their adulthood and affect their future families. Domestic violence experts find that children who are exposed to violence and intimidation suffer a range of serious problems.

- Symptoms of posttraumatic stress including depression, anxiety, and suicidal thoughts
- Sleep disorders
- Psychosomatic complaints
- Personality problems
- Conduct disorders such as acting out violently with peers
- School problems
- Poor social skills

Many men who batter women also batter their children and use them as a way to control their mothers when other methods fail. According to experts, 40 to 70% of abused children have mothers who are battered.

Jenny was caught in such a situation. Her husband knew she was afraid he would physically hurt the kids, especially her daughter. He knew she was terrified of losing custody and being seen as a bad mother. It was a horrible dilemma. She endured her husband's abuse as a way to protect herself and her kids. At the same time, she feared being found unfit in a custody dispute because she didn't adequately protect her children from their father.

Children's best interests are served by ending the entrapment that is typical of an abusive situation in which the whole family is held hostage to the abuser's efforts to control his or her mate. Children need nurturing parents, and you cannot truly attend to the emotional well-being of your children if your own psychological and physical security are compromised. Furthermore, your children will suffer from seeing and hearing the abuse.

GETTING HELP FROM THE POLICE: GOOD NEWS/BAD NEWS

Again, the picture is mixed. Some people think that in the past decade, police departments have been doing a much better job of investigating, disciplining, and terminating abusive officers. Others aren't so sure. Clearly there has been progress and increased awareness of the problem. In 2003 the International Association of Chiefs of Police (IACP) wrote a model policy for handling acts of domestic violence committed by police officers. (See the Bibliography for references to this document.) The bad news, according to the National Center for Women and Policing, is that with some notable exceptions, too few agencies are doing anything more than adding the policy to their manuals. Investigation and enforcement may still be spotty. In the 1999 study of the Baltimore Police Department, approximately 80% of the cases of police domestic abuse that were reported to the internal affairs division were dropped for lack of corroborating evidence. I don't know why this was and it may be unique to that city, but I doubt it. Victims often abandon their charges out of fear, intimidation, concerns about loss of income and health insurance, or a sincere but naive, belief that things will get better.

The Omnibus Consolidated Appropriations Act of 1997 mandates that anyone convicted of misdemeanor or felony domestic violence may not possess or use a firearm, including cops. If a cop can't use a gun, he or she can't work. Unfortunately, there are loopholes in the law, and it may be inconsistently applied. Some people are concerned that the threat of job loss has made victims even more reluctant to report being abused. Who knows what troubles await a victim whose complaints cost his or her partner a prized job?

The Omnibus Act has raised new challenges. Some departments have seen an increase in bogus abuse complaints that are being filed solely, they believe, to gain advantage in divorce actions or custody disputes. And police officers who are victims of partner abuse report that they are reluctant to defend themselves for fear of losing their jobs.

Prior to the passage of the Omnibus Act, many police agencies were taking active steps to deal with the problem, recognizing that police officers must behave humanely if they are to be effective in the community. (There are studies that suggest that police officers who are violent at home are less apt to arrest abusers and more apt to respond with hostility to victims, thus failing their basic mission to protect and serve and exposing their departments to liability.) Several big-city police departments have programs for police families in which domestic abuse occurs. The Chicago Police Department, for example, has an Office of the Domestic Violence Advocate to encourage abused spouses and partners of police officers to step forward and report abuse in the home. These departments have a top-down policy that lets officers know that domestic violence will not be tolerated. If domestic abuse occurs off duty or in another jurisdiction, it is still considered department business, not a personal family problem to be swept under the rug. With various degrees of success, these departments use some or all of the following tactics.

- Require officers involved in *any* police action to notify their command staff, thereby bringing offending officers who live in other jurisdictions to the attention of their departments. (Unfortunately, there is typically no procedure in place to ensure that courts notify police departments when a protective order is in effect. Relying on a police officer to personally inform his department of the order probably limits its effectiveness.)
- Investigate all allegations of domestic abuse: stalking, harassment, even complaints of pain without obvious bruising.
- Mandate any cop identified as a victim or perpetrator of misdemeanor domestic violence to receive counseling.
- File complaints of domestic abuse with internal affairs and use these as leverage to involve officers in counseling.
- Offer counseling: individual, family, couple, anger management, and same-sex groups.
- Remove the offending officers' weapons; put them on light duty; fine, suspend, demote, place on probation or administrative leave, or restrict overtime until allegations are resolved.
- File administrative, as well as criminal, charges.

- Utilize special domestic violence units to investigate complaints of officer-involved domestic abuse rather than leaving this to the cop's friends and beat partners.
- Provide protective custody to the victim, and take responsibility to prevent a repeat assault.

Realistically, these well-intended programs, like many programs for treating batterers, vary in effectiveness because batterers are resistant to help, persist in denying the seriousness of their actions, and can enlist the collusion of their fellow cops or superiors.

As I said earlier, victims may be reluctant to ask for help because they risk retaliation, as well as economic disaster, if their officer is disciplined or fired. Victims also resist asking for help because the help they have previously requested and received has been ineffective or created worse problems. Sometimes they are hesitant because they feel ashamed and incorrectly blame themselves for their abuse.

When abuse victims themselves are cops, male or female, they may avoid asking for support because they can't bear to think of themselves in the same category as the domestic assault victims they see at work. They may minimize the violence because it is not as bad as what they see on the job or because they are ashamed not to be able to defend themselves and control their mates.

After talking to abused spouses, researchers, and advocates, I am especially concerned about families living in small towns or rural areas. While there may be fewer cases of abuse in these small towns, as reported earlier, these victims are in a particularly tough situation. The people to whom they turn for help—other cops, doctors, judges, and lawyers—may be longtime close friends or relatives who are reluctant to take official action against each other. I've heard many stories about officers who seem superficially eager to help but then lose vital evidence or take too long to file or investigate a complaint.

Some victims may be pressured to drop charges by a close-knit group of family and friends whose religious or social values run counter to their best interests. Their officer may hold one of few steady, well-paying jobs in the area and be widely regarded in the community as a good provider and citizen. These victims may be emotionally blackmailed because of this—complain against your spouse, and he'll lose his job and his community standing. To escape and find help, a woman may have to leave her own small town—everyone and everything she knows—and risk social isolation and economic deprivation by hiding in an urban area.

STAYING SAFE

When violence occurs in your home and you have the slightest reason to think it could happen again, you need a safety plan. It is not necessary to make any decisions about separation or divorce. In fact, it is wise to take time to consider the future of your relationship. But you need a safe, calm atmosphere in which to do such serious thinking. A domestic violence advocate can help you think about and write up a safety plan, as can friends, family, coworkers, church members, and ministers. Involving trusted people in your plan is the first step in breaking the isolation that is part of the pattern of abuse.

Here's what goes into a safety plan:

- Find a phone you or your kids can use in an emergency.
- Teach your children how to call 911. Make sure they know their own address and phone number.
- Memorize or keep a list of emergency phone numbers: police, fire, and domestic violence hotline. If it seems safe to do so, program these numbers into the speed-dialing function on your phone.
- Keep change handy for making emergency calls from a pay phone.
- Choose a code word or phrase to let your kids, your friends, or your family know you need them to call the police.
- Put some money aside for an emergency.
- Think about where you and your children would go if you had to leave in a hurry, how you would get there, how long you would stay, and what would prompt you to return.
- Talk to your children about the possibility of leaving;

choose a code word to use as a signal if you need to depart quickly.

- Keep a spare set of car keys and house keys.
- Keep some money, a change of clothes, and important papers in an accessible but private place where you can get them quickly.
- Get additional information from the organizations and websites listed in the Resources section that are dedicated to domestic violence prevention.

Keeping yourself safe from violence is only the tip of the iceberg. You also need to formulate your thinking about other forms of coercion and control. Since everyone is different, the first step to take is to establish your own bottom line about what you can and cannot tolerate, including violence. If you have trouble doing this, confront what may be stopping you from taking action by listing all your fears and problem solving them one by one.

The point is that ultimately you need to decide for yourself what steps you would surely, though sorrowfully, take if an intolerable action occurred.

One way to do this and make it real for yourself is to write out a contract and stick to it. Ideally, you would share this contract with your partner. If it is not safe to do so, show it to a friend, a domestic abuse advocate, or a coworker. If you can't show it to anyone else, read it yourself every day. The following sample comes from a book by domestic violence experts Peter Neidig and Dale Friedman (1984) about treating couples for spouse abuse.

> This contract represents the action I am fully prepared to take should the behavior specified occur. This is a statement of fact, not a threat. It will be taken because it is the proper response to violence [or other abuse] and ultimately in the best interest of us all. Should these behaviors occur [list them], I will always respond by [list the actions you will take]. (pp. 205–207)

Tips for Dealing with Domestic Abuse

- Establish a zero-tolerance policy for violence of any sort in your family.
- Stop verbal abuse before it escalates.
- Don't deny the abuse—name it for what it is. It is the abuser's responsibility to control his or her own behavior, even in stressful or provocative situations. Substance abuse is not an excuse for violence, it is a reason to seek treatment.
- Contact your local domestic violence advocate or women's center. They can provide you with shelter, legal advice, and psychological support. They may know who in your spouse's department is trustworthy and reliable. They will help you get an order of protection, which, among other actions, may result in the judge's order to your spouse to surrender his or her firearm.
- Call your local domestic abuse hotline or the toll-free national hotline at 800-799-SAFE. These confidential services provide support and information.
- If your spouse's police department or other local authorities won't take action, go to the prosecuting attorney or another county for help. As a last resort, contact federal authorities for help in protecting your civil rights.
- Don't work with a therapist or advocate who insists that you must leave the relationship, that he or she knows what's best for you, or that you should discuss *your* issues, *your* anger, and so on to the exclusion of discussing your concerns about safety.
- If you fight back in defense, you take a risk that your abuser will retaliate with more violence, and you may be injured. Everyone's situation is different. Only you can decide.

CHAPTER 10

ALCOHOL ABUSE AND SUICIDE

How can officers, knowing and seeing on a daily
basis what alcohol does to citizens . . . and to
criminals, continue to drink knowing that alcohol is
far more likely to kill them than a bullet?
—SALLY GROSS-FARINA, JD,
"Fit for Duty?: Cops, Choirpractice
and Another Chance for Healing"

The other day I received a call from a newspaper reporter. He
cited two recent, highly publicized police scandals involving alcohol. "How big a problem is this?" he asked me. "Is alcoholism
more common in the police than in other occupations?" I told
him I couldn't answer that question with any accuracy because
there are no reliable statistics comparing one occupation with another in rates of alcoholism. I told him that in the United States,
approximately 1 in 10 adults in the general population is an alcoholic, and some experts think the rate for police officers is more
than double that.

What I was *really* thinking was "What difference does it
make how many there are? The crucial question is what do we
do about it? How can we get help to those officers who are
alcoholics or problem drinkers, and how can we prevent others
from following in their footsteps? How can we help their families?"

DUKE'S STORY

After I hung up the phone, I thought about Duke. Duke and I had met under pretty drastic circumstances. He was at home, drunk, angry, and yelling at the top of his lungs, prompting a neighbor to call 911. His department asked two of his closest cop friends and me to assess the situation and make a recommendation about what to do next.

Duke lived in a tiny, shabby house in a rundown neighborhood, far below the standard of living a veteran cop could afford if he wasn't paying alimony and child support to two former wives and drinking the rest. There was hardly enough furniture for four people to sit down.

We were there for hours while Duke alternately ranted or sank into morose silence. Outside, his son and some worried friends paced anxiously in the driveway. Duke was enraged at his superiors and recited a long litany of departmental injustices. He seemed to think it was *his* responsibility to right all these "wrongs," and he wanted to do so by shooting the offending administrators. He was very drunk and very dangerous.

Duke's friends and I managed to persuade him that he needed help for his drinking and his depression. We hoped he would consent to voluntarily enter a psychiatric hospital. While we were prepared to commit him, we knew that that would be the end of his career. We also knew that alcoholism is a treatable disease, and given the right care and organizational support, Duke could recover and return to work.

As is so often the case, Duke's drinking was an open secret. Many people in his department knew he had a problem with alcohol, though few understood how deeply depressed he was or the extent to which alcohol had penetrated his life and affected his family. He was widely regarded as an excellent cop, and coworkers assumed that his drinking didn't affect him at work. He was a man's man—a physically strong guy who hunted, fished, and womanized. Hard drinking just completed the picture. No one knew about the times he urinated on the floor or vomited in the hallway because he was too drunk to find the bathroom—or the blackouts, or the drunken binges.

ALCOHOLISM: MYTHS AND REALITIES

Duke's story, though drastic, is not all that unique, and it illustrates some of the myths and realities surrounding alcoholics and alcoholism.

Myth: Once an alcoholic, always an alcoholic.

Reality: Alcoholism is a disease for which recovery is guaranteed *if* the alcoholic begins and sticks with a recovery program. If not, what's guaranteed is a premature death.

Myth: Alcoholism is caused by a lack of willpower, immorality, weak character, or police stress.

Reality: No one really knows what drives a person to drink. Studies have alternately implicated physical, genetic, psychological, environmental, and social factors.

Myth: All alcoholics are skid-row drunks.

Reality: Many alcoholics hold high-level jobs and function well at work for years before their performance is noticeably affected by drinking.

Myth: If an alcoholic can stop drinking, he or she doesn't have a problem.

Reality: Abstinence is not a sign that someone is free of alcoholism. Alcoholics Anonymous (AA) calls these abstainers "dry drunks" because they have no real understanding of their condition, no new ways to cope, and are almost certain to fall off the wagon.

Myth: Alcoholics drink every day.

Reality: Alcohol abuse patterns vary. Some people get drunk daily, and others only on the weekends. Some stay sober for months and then go on a long binge.

WHAT ABOUT YOU?

Teaching "I Love a Cop" classes, I grew accustomed to hearing whispered rumors about cops' wives who were impaired by alcohol. Joan, a young wife, confided in me about her friend Ruth, who was married to a cop for 20 years. Joan worried that Ruth was becoming withdrawn and suspected she drank too much and had an unhappy, though stable, marriage. She wondered what to do and asked if I could help. Joan had asked Ruth to come to class with her, but Ruth had refused, saying her husband probably wouldn't approve. Joan was frustrated by her friend's resignation and passivity toward life. She was also frustrated by her inability to help and the fact that I discouraged her from helping Ruth sneak out of the house or lie about her whereabouts.

I never did meet Ruth, though I thought about her and others like her a lot. Studies suggest that cops' spouses, particularly those whose mates are burned out, are vulnerable to using alcohol to cope with the strain of living with someone who is unable to provide adequate emotional support, companionship, or help with parenting.

Regardless of the hardships of police relationships, using alcohol to deal with life's problems will only compound your troubles. Although you may be reading this chapter out of concern for someone else, think, too, of your own health and well-being; consider your own drinking habits, as well as those of your loved one.

SIGNS AND SYMPTOMS OF ALCOHOL ABUSE

In the first edition of *I Love a Cop*, I included the following checklist, adapted from the National Council on Alcoholism and the Kaiser Permanente Medical Care Program, as a rough estimate to determine whether you or someone close to you may need help with his or her drinking. Since then I have discovered a checklist specifically designed for police officers. You can find it in the "Tips for Dealing with the Problem-Drinking Cop" on pages 193–194.

Yes	No		Is This You?
(circle one)			
Y	N	1.	Have you ever felt the need or tried to cut down on your alcohol intake?
Y	N	2.	Do you test yourself for control, say you won't drink, and then take a drink anyway?

Y N 3. Do you think it would be difficult to enjoy life if you could not take another drink?

Y N 4. Do you use alcohol as a way of handling stressful situations or life problems?

Y N 5. Have you ever gotten angry at someone for telling you that you drink too much?

Y N 6. Have you ever felt guilty about your drinking?

Y N 7. Have you ever felt as if you needed a drink to get going in the morning?

Y N 8. Do you hide your alcohol or drink secretly?

Y N 9. Do you take more drinks than you had planned?

Y N 10. Do you have wide swings in mood and personality?

Y N 11. Can you drink more than you used to?

Y N 12. Do you ever wake up the morning after and find you can't remember part of the evening before?

Y N 13. Do you feel uncomfortable if alcohol is not readily available?

Y N 14. Are you in more of a hurry to get that first drink?

Y N 15. Do you regret things you have done or said while drinking?

Y N 16. Are you having an increasing number of financial, family, sexual, or work problems because of alcohol?

Y N 17. Do you eat irregularly or very little when you are drinking?

Y N 18. Have you had any legal problems, for example a DUI [driving under the influence] arrest, related to your use of alcohol?

Y N 19. Do you sometimes get the "shakes" in the morning and find it helps to have a little drink?

Y N 20. Do you regularly use over-the-counter medications and/or prescription drugs to counteract alcohol-induced insomnia, stomach distress, headaches, or hangovers?

If you answered yes to one or more items, you or your mate should think seriously about getting help.

Note about drug use. Many alcoholics also abuse drugs, most often over-the-counter medications or prescription drugs. Of course, there are cops who use illegal drugs, but police departments don't tolerate illegal drug abusers in the same way they tolerate known alcoholics or problem drinkers. Concerns about liability have increased over the past decade. Some enlightened police departments still offer rehabilitation and full or modified employment to the recovering alcoholic, but it is rare to find a department that will offer the same to a cop who is recovering from addiction to an illegal substance.

RISK FACTORS FOR COPS

I wish I could talk to that reporter who was interested in knowing how many alcoholic cops there are compared to alcoholism in other professions. Now, instead of talking numbers, I'd like to talk about risk factors. Cops have the same risk factors as those in other hard-drinking, nonpolice occupations—high levels of job stress, peer pressure, isolation from the mainstream, a preponderance of young males and a culture that approves of using alcohol to relax and cope with stress.

But cops also have some unique risks. Hazardous habits such as a need for emotional control combined with a disposition mentality—solve the problem and move on—make cops eager to get rid of their problems rather than face them or work through them. Hypervigilance drives cops to seek extreme means to kick back and relax. Image armor and the myth that cops are problem-free problem solvers encourage relying on booze, as well as people, to reduce stress and tension. Alcohol abuse in emergency responders at the 1995 Oklahoma City bombing was the second most reported coping strategy after seeking interpersonal support. There are similar reports following other catastrophic events; the more vulnerable the person was before the trauma, the higher the risk of substance abuse afterward.

The psychological and biographical factors that press people into police work add to the risk, especially the need to feel invincible and a corresponding longing for the perfect family of invincible protectors. Duke's rage at his administrators for being inadequate, as well as his disregard for his own physical and emotional limits, illustrate that all too common dynamic.

Finally, the widely held notion that many cops come from alcoholic families may mean that some are at risk for abusing alcohol because they have a genetic predisposition or vulnerability to alcoholism.

COVER-UPS AND COLLUSIONS

Some people collude with alcoholics: They do things to help the drinker cover his or her mistakes or minimize his or her responsibility— often while simultaneously protesting the drinker's behavior. This is popularly referred to as "enabling" or codependency. On the other hand, it is apparent that certain so-called collusive actions are necessary because some families are dependent on the alcoholic breadwinner.

This is Irma's predicament. Irma has to take over the bill paying because Durk, her husband, gets drunk and forgets to pay the bills on time more often than he remembers. Is Irma covering up for him by not confronting his irresponsibility, or is she looking after her family and fighting to hold on to their possessions? This is a difficult question to answer, and the answer may be different for every family.

The most frequent way in which cops collude with each other is to cover up alcohol-related misconduct until there is a crisis, at which point they may disown the officer they have protected and tolerated for years. Cops cover up alcoholic misconduct in a lot of ways: They don't arrest a coworker they have stopped for driving under the influence; they don't ticket an illegally parked car that belongs to a drunken cop; they drive when their partner is too hungover to navigate and wants to sleep it off in the back seat; they ignore the smell of booze on an on-duty coworker's breath; they talk spouses and lovers out of reporting alcohol-related violence; or they rationalize the theft of drugs from evidence because cops need them, deserve them, and have even "earned" the right to use them to stay awake on long surveillances. Attorney Sally Gross-Farina, former cop and police therapist, believes that cops love the idea that they alone love each other and will protect each other against all outsiders. Is it in this spirit that they run union-sponsored police-only bars and hold social functions where they can get plastered without running into the public? How absurd to think that cops are so invincible that they can encourage each other to get drunk but not to be drunks.

OBSTACLES TO GETTING HELP

A police officer might not want to get help for many reasons, the primary one being that he or she isn't ready to give up drinking. But other considerations are unique to the profession. Police officers can never predict when they might run into someone they know at an AA meeting: a person they have arrested, a defendant against whom they're scheduled to testify, or someone who could blow their undercover identity.

When police officers are apprehensive about revealing what they do for a living, it can inhibit their ability to speak openly and compromise their treatment. If they do tell people they are cops, it might compromise their safety.

Are these concerns realistic, or are they excuses to continue drinking? This probably depends on the person and his or her circumstances. I prefer to regard them as challenges that can be managed by utilizing some of the tips at the end of this section.

WHAT'S A FAMILY TO DO?

Families of alcoholics are usually desperate and have tried all sorts of strategies to deal with their problem drinkers. They've monitored their drinking, hidden their booze, cleaned up after them, held their heads, held their hands, left them, took them back, yelled, pleaded, threatened, cried, reasoned, thrown things, blamed their job, blamed their friends, or blamed themselves in a frenzy of unsuccessful attempts to save the drinker and save the family. Often such desperation occurs in a stifling atmosphere of secrecy and pretense, where no one in the family feels safe enough to talk about what is *really* going on at home and how everyone feels about it.

A support group, individual counseling, or family therapy can help you and your family deal with the emotional strain of living with an alcoholic and the delicate process of constructing a life with or without your mate. You can determine if you are sufficiently concerned about someone's drinking to profit from support or counseling by answering this 20-question quiz from Al-Anon.

Y N   1. Do you worry about how much someone else drinks?

Y N   2. Do you have money problems because of someone else's drinking?

Y N   3. Do you tell lies to cover up for someone else's drinking?

Y N   4. Do you feel that if the drinker loved you, he or she would stop drinking to please you?

Y N   5. Do you blame the drinker's behavior on his or her companions?

Y N   6. Are plans frequently upset or canceled or meals delayed because of the drinker?

Y N   7. Do you make threats, such as "If you don't stop drinking, I'll leave you"?

Y N   8. Do you secretly try to smell the drinker's breath?

Y N   9. Are you afraid to upset someone for fear it will set off a drinking bout?

Y N   10. Have you been hurt or embarrassed by a drinker's behavior?

Y N   11. Are holidays and gatherings spoiled because of drinking?

Y N   12. Have you considered calling the police for help in fear of abuse?

Y N   13. Do you search for hidden alcohol?

Y N   14. Do you often ride in a car with a driver who has been drinking?

Y N   15. Have you refused social invitations out of fear or anxiety?

Y N   16. Do you sometimes feel like a failure when you think of the lengths you have gone to control the drinker?

Y   N   17. Do you think that if the drinker stopped drinking, your other problems would be solved?

Y   N   18. Do you ever threaten to hurt yourself to scare the drinker?

Y   N   19. Do you feel angry, confused, or depressed most of the time?

Y   N   20. Do you feel no one understands your problems?

If you answered yes to three or more questions, you may find Al-Anon, some other support group, or counseling to be invaluable to you and to your family.

Step Back

As part of a public safety family, you may have a little of that take-charge, take-action attitude that cops have. For this reason, you're probably more at risk for doing too much rather than doing too little, especially if you have gotten used to pinch hitting or doing it all because you can no longer rely on your mate. If you grew up in a family in which one or both of your parents had a drinking problem, you may fall into this take-charge, take-action attitude by sheer force of habit.

You can start by going online and learning all you can about alcoholism and/or the experience of growing up in an alcoholic family. At the same time, you can see what local resources are available for yourself and your children—libraries are gold mines of useful information. Also check both your own and your mate's health benefits to see if your family is entitled to prepaid counseling. (Chapter 11 will help you with these choices.)

Next you will need to turn your attention away from the alcoholic toward yourself—a process Al-Anon calls "releasing." What this allows you to do is release the alcoholic to make his or her own choice to continue drinking or to stop. Stepping back may feel uncomfortable, as if you are abandoning your loved one. Keep in mind that because alcoholism is a disease that affects the whole family, when any family member changes his or her behavior, it may spur the alcoholic toward recovery. Stepping back may actually be more productive than all the pleading, bargaining, threatening, or arguing you have tried in the past.

What does it mean to step back? Here's what it meant to Millie, who for years had struggled with her husband, Howard, over his drinking. First Millie decided *she* had to change because Howard wouldn't or couldn't, even though he tried. Each time he failed, they were both devastated. Millie decided that although she didn't want to leave Howard, she could no longer afford to ride this emotional roller coaster with him. She resolved to take a position of noninvolvement, not rejection. She literally taught herself to regard Howard's relationship to alcohol with detachment, compassion, and patience. She took up yoga and meditation to support her determination to stay calm and detached.

Millie stopped giving advice, rescuing, nagging, or reacting. This in itself helped since what either one of them said or did in anger often made matters worse. She no longer woke Howard when he slept through the alarm; she took her own car to social events; she went ahead with dinner whether Howard was home from work or not. All of this was very scary to Millie. But she stuck it out because she knew from experience that accommodating Howard's drinking hadn't helped either of them.

Things got rockier at home; Howard became morose and accused Millie of not caring about him. Oddly enough, Millie was feeling better than she had in years. Her self-esteem was up, and she felt stronger and more adult. Howard tried to get Millie to change back to her old ways and eventually gave up in a funk. He went to a few AA meetings and stopped when she didn't react, other than to be calmly supportive. Recently he has started going again.

One important step Millie took was to address the problem directly, taking Howard's drinking for what it was rather than pretending that he was sick, sleepy, overmedicated, and so on. More than once Millie and the kids had kept on eating after Howard had passed out at the table. They told each other he was tired and fell asleep.

There are a lot of reasons that families of alcoholics don't talk honestly about what is happening in their midst—shame, loyalty, uncertainty, mistrust, fear of the consequences, and so on. This sets an example that kids may carry for life, damaging *their* adult relationships.

Set Your Bottom Line

According to Dr. Harriet Lerner, setting a bottom line means you figure out what is and isn't acceptable to you in regard to your loved one's drinking. Once you establish your bottom line, stick to it—empty threats are useless. Reread Chapter 9 for ideas about making contracts describing how you will respond to those actions you consider intolerable. Even though alcoholism is a disease, it does not absolve the alcoholic from responsibility for his or her choices, including the choice to drink.

Establishing your bottom line will also help you stand up to a number of challenges. Family and friends may want you to be the way you used to be and will test your resolve. Dealing with their "change-back" messages and countermoves takes guts and energy. Having a bottom line will also help you prepare for relapses, if they occur, and for resolving family problems that have been ignored because everyone was so focused on the drinker and his or her problems.

Being immersed in a drinker's behavior makes it easy to lose track of the plans you have made for yourself and your family. Setting a bottom line helps you to get back on track. We all have issues larger than whether our mates do or do not drink. We all need to consider our futures, figure out who we are and what we stand for, get involved in activities that stimulate us, care for our families and our communities, find meaningful work, and earn enough money to provide ourselves with a decent standard of living.

It is misleading to think that things will be perfect if and when the alcoholic stops drinking. Recovery from alcoholism is a long-haul project with many ups and downs. AA and other 12-step programs say the process never ends. They encourage alcoholics to make a lifetime commitment to a recovery program.

Tips for Dealing with the Problem-Drinking Cop

Tell your cop about this checklist—don't nag or force the issue; just offer the resource.

Twenty Questions for Cops (adapted with permission from Dr. Craig Weissman, Los Angeles Sheriff's Department)

Y N 1. Have you ever called in sick the day after a training party because you were too hungover to function?

Y N 2. Do you take pride in being able to function after drinking more than any of your friends?

Y N 3. Have you ever called up an ex-spouse or lover at the end of a night of heavy drinking?

Y N 4. Do you regularly stop for a drink on the way home to calm down before you face your family?

Y N 5. Do your coworkers ever tease you about your behavior while drinking?

Y N 6. While working dogwatch, do you ever drink at the end of your shift, rationalizing that it was really the end of your day?

Y N 7. Have you ever been so drunk at a department party that it seemed like a good idea to tell off one of the brass?

Y N 8. Do you start drinking before you go to functions where alcohol is being served?

Y N 9. Do you check with your friends to see if you did anything stupid because you cannot remember what you did while you were drinking?

Y N 10. Do you mistrust cops who do not drink as much as you do?

Y N 11. When you stop drinking, do you feel shaky and have a hard time sleeping?

Y N 12. If your coworkers were asked, "Who is the heaviest drinker here?" would they all look in your direction?

Y N 13. When drinking, have you ever shown somebody your gun to persuade them to see things your way? *(cont.)*

(continued from previous page)

Y N 14. Are you sharing your hard-earned money with an ex-spouse because your drinking behavior led to the end of your marriage?

Y N 15. Have you ever damaged your car or motorcycle when driving after drinking?

Y N 16. The morning after a night of heavy drinking, have you ever looked over at the person lying next to you and realized you made a terrible mistake?

Y N 17. Has a coworker ever commented that you smell of alcohol at work?

Y N 18. Do you think these questions were rigged to make you look like you have a drinking problem?

Y N 19. Has a doctor ever suggested that you quit drinking or at least cut down?

Y N 20. Have you ever been told to go to Peace Officer Fellowship meetings or AA?

If your officer is concerned about his or her safety and anonymity and this is keeping him or her from getting help, refer him or her to the following tips offered by recovering officers:

- Contact your employee assistance program and ask for a cops-only meeting, sometimes known as the Peace Officer's Fellowship (California and Pennsylvania), No Cops Out (Illinois), or Bottles and Badges (New York).
- Find a peer supporter or a sponsor who is a cop in recovery.
- Find a residential program that does not use second offender funding or other criminal justice diversion funds and is priced to screen out some criminal elements but not cops.
- Start at AA by going to Speaker's Meetings or Step Studies, where you will not be expected to reveal personal information.
- For your first meetings, pretend you are working undercover. Speak in a general way until you get comfortable. If

you know other cops in the group, pay attention to what they do or don't say.

SUICIDE

Suicide among police officers is a dramatic example of what happens when those entrusted with the protection of others fail to protect and care for themselves.
—SGT. MICHAEL TIGHE, *NYPD*

How does a person who was once hardy enough to pass a demanding application process, a rigorous psychological screening, and an arduous training program become so overwhelmed that suicide is his only out? How does a professional problem solver get so low that suicide seems to be the best solution to her problems? There are probably as many reasons and combinations of reasons as there are officers who kill themselves.

For years, police professionals and mental health professionals have tried to reconstruct events that lead to suicide. Their psychological autopsies implicate alcoholism, family conflicts, relationship losses, disciplinary problems, depression, immediate access to guns and skill in using them, drug abuse, poor coping skills, financial difficulties, age and gender, job stress, scandal, shame, failure, and a distorted but culturally correct sense of invincibility and independence. If there is a common thread linking these elements, it is the doomed officer's inability to ask for or find confidential help before small problems snowball into a tidal wave of torment.

How big a problem is this? Similar to divorce statistics, statistics about the frequency of suicide among police officers are inconclusive because there is no systematic way to collect accurate data connecting suicide to occupation. Some people think that the numbers are artificially low, as cops may try to cover up a suicide out of pride and a desire to protect the surviving family from losing their insurance benefits. But, I, as well as most of my colleagues, think estimates of police suicide have been artificially inflated, the result of making an inappropriate comparison between police officers and the general population. When you compare police officers to white males between the ages of 21 and 55, which represents the majority of police officers, you find that law enforcement personnel are 26% less likely to commit suicide than their same-sex, -race, and -age civilian counterparts.

It is also a popular belief, one I included in the previous edition of this chapter, that cops are more likely to kill themselves than be killed in the line of duty. Current views seem to support this as a reliable, though not exact, calculation.

In the years between 2002 and 2005, an average of 151 officers died in the line of duty. Knowing what we do about the rate of suicide among the police (18.1 per 100,000 officers), an estimated average of 122 officers would have killed themselves during that same time period.

It is my contention that these more accurate numbers will help dispel frightening and discouraging myths, but I know that numbers are neither consoling nor helpful when someone you know is contemplating suicide.

Joe is a good example of how mounting problems can push an officer to the brink of suicide and how timely intervention can pull him back. Joe had been an alcoholic for years. His poor work performance finally caught up to him when a young, energetic supervisor replaced his former sergeant, who had been a friend and a drinking buddy. The new sergeant began to pressure Joe to be more productive and read all his reports carefully, kicking most of them back for errors. Then he disciplined Joe for an improper traffic stop and warned him that he faced harsher discipline and possible termination if he didn't bring his work up to acceptable standards. When Joe made another serious mistake, he was told he would be given two days off and mandated to ride with a field training officer for a month of remedial training. Joe felt humiliated and exposed by this mandate. He raged at the supervisor and threatened to file a grievance.

At the same time, his wife, Margaret, had come to the end of her patience with Joe's drinking. Joe wasn't violent, and he didn't run around. He just wasn't there for her, and he would fall asleep after dinner every night and on the weekends. They hardly talked to each other, and they had no social life. Their sex life was nonexistent.

Losing Margaret and facing serious work problems drove Joe into a state of despair. He felt absolutely powerless to improve his circumstances, and he saw no options. He didn't know how to stop drinking and was convinced he would lose his job or have his gun taken from him if he went to the department psychologist for help (there were rumors that the psychologist blabbed everything to the chief). Joe didn't feel he could muster the energy he needed to satisfy his supervisor, and he couldn't figure out how to make it up with Margaret, or even if he wanted to. He was depressed and angry at himself and everyone else around him. Mostly he felt lost and helpless.

At first, Joe thought briefly about suicide; then he began to consider it seriously as an option. He was so overwhelmed that the idea developed from a better option to, finally, what appeared to be his only option. One night he couldn't bear going home to an empty house so he sat in his car in the station parking lot and put his gun in his mouth. He didn't have time to let the feelings of despair subside because his gun was right there on the seat next to him. A couple of other cops saw him, smashed through the window, and yanked his gun away.

This close call brought Joe the attention he needed. He was placed on administrative leave while he received treatment for alcoholism and depression. Three years later he returned to full duty and worked until his retirement. He and Margaret were divorced. Help came too late to save his marriage but not too late to save his life and his job.

Red Flags/Warning Signs

Most people who commit suicide give hints—some clear, some coded—that suicide is on their mind or that they are deeply distressed about something. Every item in the following discussion is an indication that a person needs help, whether or not that person is actively considering suicide.

Serious Depression

Serious depression is more than a case of the blues. Depressed people have a hopeless, pessimistic outlook on life. They may be anxious, bitter, irritable, restless, and underfunctioning. They are withdrawn and get little or no joy out of life or the things that once pleased them. Seriously depressed people have trouble sleeping and may have no appetite or sex drive. They may be lethargic and often sick; they may lose weight and take little interest in their appearance. You may or may not be able to see what caused their depression; sometimes it is obvious—like a death in the family—and sometimes it is not.

Depressed people may be inwardly punitive, filled with guilt, shame, and self-hatred. It is almost as though they have a double life—they appear to be adjusted and successful, but they secretly feel like impostors. The strain of covering up or the fear of exposing their inadequacies can precipitate a suicide attempt.

While a great many suicidal people are clinically depressed, they are only rarely psychotic. More than likely their distress results from a tangled series of events and a temporarily hopeless outlook. Even if they are clinically depressed or suffering from some emotional disability, depression and mental illness are treatable with medication and psychotherapy. The common element in suicide is hopelessness and/or helplessness, not mental illness.

A Significant Loss—Actual or Threatened

We will all suffer losses in our lives: loss of friends, family, health, pride, looks, love, confidence, money, work, reputation, dreams, and so on. Everyone copes differently with loss, and every loss is different. Some losses mount up or occur in a series. Many people, especially cops, push themselves to recover from a loss before they are ready. Sometimes this comes back to haunt them later on.

Cops who lose their jobs because of an injury face a double whammy. They have lost health and vigor, as well as an identity, a purpose in life, and fraternity. This kind of transition stirs up significant emotional turmoil, and cops need a lot of support during this time, especially if they feel retirement has been forced on them by medical doctors or administrators.

Unfortunately, many cops ignore the serious emotional losses that go with premature retirement. They laugh it off—perhaps to avoid thinking it could happen to them too—and kid the retiree about faking problems and conning the employer. Some folks envy and greatly overrate the disabled cop's tax-free income, and it keeps them from seeing things through the retiree's eyes. Many cops I know who retired prematurely wind up being happier than they have been in ages. Still, there may be a rocky transition while they are adjusting to the idea and worrying about future unknowns.

The loss of a relationship is perhaps the most devastating loss, one that is frequently associated with suicide. It is sadly ironic that cops who maintain an I-don't-need-you attitude toward their mates can sometimes be devastated when the one they have pushed away or kept at a distance eventually leaves.

Substance Abuse

You already know this—people who abuse drugs or alcohol are at risk for many forms of self-destructive behavior, suicide being the most serious. Uncontrolled drinking or drug abuse, along with smoking, is a slow, passive form of suicide. Some studies predict that 15% of all alcoholics will commit active suicide during their lifetimes. An angry separation or divorce will be the most common precipitating event.

Previous Suicide Attempts or Threats

It is a myth that people who threaten or attempt suicide will not actually do it. Most suicidal people are undecided about living or dying. It is rare that someone commits suicide without letting others know in advance how he or she is feeling. Unfortunately, their cry for help is often indirect and hard to decipher.

People who talk about their hopeless situation or who readily identify with the "benefits" of suicide may be debating about whether or not to end their lives. Statements such as "What's the use," "I can't live this way anymore," "They'd be better off if I were dead," and so on, even when said jokingly, should be taken seriously by others. The same is true for people who seem to be obsessed with the subject of suicide, particularly the details used in planning it.

Marked Change in Personality

Pay attention to the person whose personality seems to have changed. This could be an indication of a psychological or a physical illness.

199

Occasionally, people who have decided that suicide is their best option become deceptively happy at having made this decision. When they kill themselves, their family and friends are stunned because they thought their loved one was on the mend. A burst of energy or happiness in a despairing person or within three months of a suicidal crisis is cause for concern. Someone needs to ask this person, "Are things really better with you or have you decided to kill yourself?"

Giving Things Away

When people break off relationships or give away their personal possessions, particularly valued possessions such as a pet or a piece of jewelry, they may have decided to die. They give things away happily because they have made a decision that looks like a solution to their problems and because, in their distorted thinking, others will benefit more from their deaths than their lives.

Reckless Behavior

We all know cops who drink and drive, smoke when their doctor has forbidden it, fail to wait for backup, take on dangerous situations alone, and so on. They seem always to be courting disaster. Some of these people are natural-born thrill seekers who have a high need for excitement. But some are so ambivalent about living that they essentially leave that decision to chance or someone else. Cops who are extreme risk takers may be hoping to die in a blaze of glory or cover up their suicide so that it looks job-related. Unfortunately, some of these officers are praised for their bravery when they should be counseled about their intentions.

When Duke was planning to assassinate the management staff of his department, he knew that he would inevitably be killed in the process. A lot of suicidal cops, particularly angry ones, have this kind of death fantasy. It is a terrible tragedy, not just for the suicidal officer, but also for his or her fellow officers, who are forced into a harrowing and dangerous confrontation with one of their own.

Anniversary Reactions and Reunion Fantasies

The wish to join a loved one in death is particularly strong around a significant anniversary date. It is important to acknowledge anniversary reactions and to talk about the dead, rather than avoid the subject in the mistaken belief that it is less painful not to talk about it. This is particularly so if the officer harbors any notion that he or she was in some way responsible for the death or injury of a colleague.

Tips for Dealing with the Suicidal Cop

- Don't hesitate to speak openly about suicide. You can't put the idea in anyone's head if it isn't already there. It can clear the air to raise the issue and call it for what it is without using euphemisms. Ask directly, "Are you thinking of killing yourself, committing suicide, eating your gun?" and so on.
- Be assertive. Level with your loved one about your concerns; ask directly what is causing so much pain that he or she wants to stop living. Communicate your understanding that she is in great emotional pain, but clearly say that pain can be managed and that there are other ways to solve these problems beside suicide. Let him know that getting help is a sign of strength, not weakness, and that it takes guts to face your problems and yourself.
- Be honest in describing your own experience with depression, hopelessness, or thinking about suicide. Talk about what specifically helped you get through troubled times.
- Assess the level of danger—the more specific the plan, the more imminent and deadly. You need to know if you should call 911 right away or if you have time to do something else. For example, one suicidal cop told his partner he had picked out a motel; written a note for the motel staff, warning them to call the police before entering his room; written to his family; bought a tarp to keep his brains from splattering; and bought a rifle because he didn't want to use his duty gun. This was a dire emergency, requiring immediate intervention and hospitalization.

(cont.)

(continued from previous page)

Another cop, who was on disability leave, confessed to his wife that he was thinking about suicide but didn't want to kill himself on impulse, so he locked his weapons in a friend's gun locker and put the key in a bank safe deposit box. His wife was able to verify this. She alerted his therapist immediately, and the therapist arranged to see him the next day, increased their sessions, and arranged for a medication appointment.

- Be prepared. If you are going to confront a troubled loved one, plan in advance—have phone numbers available, take another friend along, or have someone standing by a telephone. Pick an appropriate time and place to raise your concerns—one that is private, comfortable, and unhurried. Unless the situation is urgent, as it was for Duke, it's better not to talk to someone who has been drinking.

- Prepare yourself for a lot of angry denial. Remember, cops think they should solve problems, not have them.

- Be direct, yet tactful. Unless the situation is imminently life-threatening, never back people into a corner by taking control away from them, threatening them, or delivering ultimatums. Suicidal people are already feeling out of control of their lives, and in their despair, they may believe suicide is the only way to get back into control.

- Give hope: Find out if this person has survived some past crisis. Sometimes remembering he or she has been through tough times before helps to restore confidence and hope for the future. People are generally suicidal for a limited time only, and if they avoid self-destruction, they can go on to lead productive lives. Hope is the awareness that one has options.

- There's a bumper sticker that says, "Cheer up, things could be worse. So I cheered up, and sure enough things got worse." Attempting to cheer someone up may be a well-intentioned move that is almost guaranteed to backfire. The listener may feel that you simply don't understand the depth of his or her despair. You will be written off, and the troubled cop may feel more isolated than before. Cheering up is different from giving hope.

(cont.)

- Don't worry more about someone losing his or her gun than his or her life. Without life there is no hope. Cops routinely underestimate the compassion they can expect from their administrators. Even if the administrators are punitive, no one's job is worth more than that person's life. The point is to intervene before your loved one is so desperate that someone is forced to take his or her gun.
- Intervention is the key to preventing suicide. The consequences of getting help to someone are *never* as permanent as the consequences of suicide. Having meaningful, supportive relationships and a therapeutic alliance with a mental health professional greatly reduces a person's risk for suicide.
- Don't argue with, give sermons to, or lecture to a suicidal person. Telling that person that suicide is a sin, that other people are worse off, that he or she shouldn't feel what he or she does feel, and so forth may only make the suicidal individual more defensive and make you less helpful. Try to see, in concrete terms, how and why this person has come to see things as he or she does—the suicidal individual didn't arrive at this point overnight.
- Respect your own limitations. Sometimes there is no way to stop people from killing themselves or to have read their mind beforehand. Do not make offers of help you cannot reasonably support: If you are troubled, overburdened with your own problems, or simply don't care enough about this person, your best move is to find someone who does and make a referral to a mental health professional.
- People who kill themselves are responsible for their choices. One person *cannot* drive another to suicide except under the most extreme circumstances.
- Take sufficient precautions. Remember, there are guns around.

GETTING HELP

CHAPTER 11

GETTING THE HELP YOU NEED
WHEN YOU NEED IT

Millions of Americans who might benefit from
psychotherapy never even give it a try. . . . That's a
shame. . . . Four thousand of our readers . . . sought
help . . . for psychological problems. . . . The
majority were highly satisfied with the care they
received. Most had made strides toward resolving the
problems that led to treatment, and almost all said
life had become more manageable.
—*CONSUMER REPORTS*, November 1995

I was surprised and happy to find an article about psychotherapy
in *Consumer Reports* (November 1995): that venerable, neutral,
not-in-anyone's-debt-no-advertising-accepted magazine that Americans depend on for accurate ratings about everything from TV
sets to toys and blankets to booster cables. I was even happier to
find a similar report, with similar results, in 2004. Here's a summary of the most recent survey of 3,000 readers.

• People were equally satisfied and reported similar progress
whether they saw a social worker, psychologist, or psychiatrist.
• Readers who sought help from their family doctor received
mostly medication. The care received from primary-care physicians was effective for mild problems, but experts interviewed for

this survey concluded that most primary-care physicians have neither the time nor the training to diagnose or treat more severe emotional concerns.

• Talk therapy rivaled drug therapy in effectiveness. The most successful intervention was a combination of talk and drugs. But respondents whose therapy was mostly talk and lasted at least 13 sessions did nearly as well or better than those whose treatment was mostly medication.

• People whose therapy was mostly medication experienced the quickest symptom relief, but many reported side effects and said it took time to find the right medication.

• In the 1995 survey, people averaged over 20 visits with a mental health professional. In the current survey, the average was 10. Since longer-term therapy is linked to more positive outcomes, that trend is troubling, as are the frustrations many respondents experienced dealing with their insurance providers.

YES, BUT: SPECIAL CONSIDERATIONS FOR COPS

You're probably thinking that *Consumer Reports* is okay if you want to buy a lawn mower or a computer but that cops and their families have special needs when buying mental health services. You're both right and wrong. There *are* special circumstances when issues of confidentiality, the culture of policing, and liability *must* be considered; although in my opinion, many of these concerns are overrated by cops and may be used as a convenient excuse for not getting the help they need. And I am certain these professional concerns should *not* keep family members from getting help.

Cops in therapy, unless they are dealing with specific work-related events, have the same basic human concerns and needs that we all have—they want to be loved, accepted, and respected as parents, children, friends, mates, employees, and community members. They want peace of mind and self-esteem. They are no more unique than the rest of us, with our distinctive personal histories, dreams, points of view, values, challenges, strengths, and weaknesses.

CONFIDENTIALITY: WHEN YOU HAVE IT, WHEN YOU DON'T

When You Have It

Confidentiality is a big concern to *all* prospective therapy clients. Licensed mental health professionals are *required* by statute and by their professional codes of ethics and conduct—which are similar to the law enforcement code of ethics—to keep all records confidential. If they do not, they risk losing the license they need to practice, and they open themselves up to lawsuits. (See p. 212 for information on confidentiality and insurance carriers.)

Here's how it works. Confidentiality is not an inherent right but a privilege. As a psychotherapy client, you, not your therapist, hold this privilege. Therapists strongly believe that psychotherapy works only in an atmosphere of trust and safety, so they will make every effort to honor your privilege.

For instance, a cop innocently told her supervisor that she and her husband, who was also a cop, were seeing a therapist. Her supervisor called the therapist, wanting to know about the client's problems and if they would affect her ability to work. The therapist refused to talk to the supervisor, telling her that revealing anything, even whether her subordinate was a client, was illegal and unethical.

The same thing holds true for family members. My colleagues and I have all had awkward half-conversations with desperate spouses who were trying to understand why their mates were treating them coldly or wanting a separation. "Could you just say," he or she pleads, "was it me, or is there someone else? Please tell me what to do." We all feel badly for such callers, but under the circumstances, we can do nothing but refer them to a therapist of their own. We cannot even acknowledge that their spouse is our client.

When You Don't

There are some circumstances under which a therapist is required by law to break confidentiality. Depending upon where you live, these are generally the same circumstances facing other mandatory reporters such as cops, physicians, and teachers.

Imminent Threat of Violence to Self or Others

If you are a threat to yourself or someone else, the therapist has a duty to warn your intended victim and the police of your intentions.

When Duke, the alcoholic officer in Chapter 10, threatened his administrators, I was required by law to inform them of his threats. Duke was also so clearly suicidal that if he were not threatening others, I would have taken steps to commit him, and that would have required discussing his case with the staff of the admitting hospital and the police. I was also required to break confidentiality with Andy, the brain-injured officer in Chapter 4, who wanted to shoot his commander.

Therapists have a checklist to determine the severity of a client's intentions to kill him- or herself or harm others. They won't break confidentiality solely on the basis of a statement such as "I'm so mad at my wife, I could kill her." But, if an officer does say something like that, expect the therapist to take the statement seriously and ask the client about it in detail.

Abuse

If you reveal that you are physically, emotionally, or sexually abusing a child, an elderly person, and in some states your spouse, your therapist is required to report this to the appropriate protective service agency and the police.

If your child or your elderly parent tells a therapist that he or she is being abused or has been abused in the past, the therapist is required to notify the police and the appropriate protective agency.

Grave Disability

If you are so disabled that you are unable to care for yourself, your therapist is mandated to report it.

Mandatory Counseling

Cops may be mandated to see a mental health professional because of performance problems, interpersonal conflicts, critical incidents, disciplinary problems, and so forth. In some departments, counseling is part of a disciplinary diversion program; the officer is given an option to get counseling instead of discipline.

Mandatory counseling is not confidential, which is a good reason for a cop to go voluntarily before counseling is ordered. Depending upon the circumstances, sometimes the cop, the therapist, and the department can reach an agreement that allows the officer some degree of privacy.

For example, Clive was referred for counseling after a series of complaints about his badge-heavy attitude toward citizens. He was infuriated and refused to go until ordered, at which time he said he would go but not say anything. The therapist pointed out that even though Clive was ordered to come, how he used the time was up to him, and he might just get something out of it since he appeared to be at risk for getting fired unless he got a handle on his temper. To help Clive feel safer, the therapist persuaded his department that he need only report any missed appointments and that the content of what he and Clive discussed would be confidential.

Fitness-for-Duty Evaluations

There is *never* any confidentiality in a fitness-for-duty evaluation. Although laws change from state to state, in general, the scope of the written report is limited to the examiner's opinion about your mental and emotional ability to safely work as a police officer, a description of your limitations, how they may or may not be accommodated, and a determination about whether these limitations are or are not work related. The evaluating therapist should give the officer a written statement to this effect and then have the officer sign the paper, confirming that he or she understands. Family members may be asked but not required to talk to the psychologist. Whatever they say is also not confidential.

Worker's Compensation Claims

In California, as in other states, when plaintiffs in a lawsuit claim damage to their mental health, they waive any confidentiality of their mental health records, past or present.

Even if there is no lawsuit, when a cop is being treated for a work-related emotional disability, the treating therapist is required to provide the worker's compensation insurance administrator with monthly reports about the client's progress.

Therapists will discuss this requirement with their clients. Some may offer to show clients their monthly reports because it is the client's right to see their files, and worker's compensation files are public records. These reports can and should be limited to the minimum necessary information about the client's general progress.

So, if an officer is fighting with his spouse because he is in the throes of a posttraumatic stress reaction, I would say that the incident had a disturbing effect on his home life but could omit the details, that he threw his dinner on the floor, and she stomped out the door and stayed with her sister for the night.

Insurance Carriers

When medical insurance is used to pay for therapy, the insurance carrier has the right to get the information needed to process the claim. In most instances, the information is limited to a billing invoice with the dates of the sessions, the services provided, the diagnosis, and the therapist's fee. Somewhere in fine print on the insurance policy the client is forewarned about this and given a release to sign.

Peer Support and Critical Incident Debriefings

Critical incident group debriefings are not confidential even when led by a licensed professional. You can request that what is said stays in the room, but there is no guarantee.

Some states now grant privileged communication to peer supporters. But in most states police officers are cops first and peer supporters second, and they can be ordered to give information. Generally, administrators recognize the value of peer support and group debriefings and do what they can to avoid intruding or putting people in uncomfortable positions. Just to be cautious, the limits of confidentiality should be explicitly stated in the department's general orders and should be reviewed in initial peer support contacts and at the beginning of a group debriefing.

Supervision, Consultation, and Cocktail Parties

Do shrinks talk about clients behind their backs? Therapists consult with supervisors and peers. They present "cases" without full names or identifying details. This is a form of professional development for the therapist that leads to quality assurance for the client. It is very different from careless gossip about clients, which is unethical and can result in censure for the offender.

Because therapists work behind closed doors, it is easy to hide professional deficits. A mental health professional who engages in ongoing training, seeks guidance about difficult cases, and operates within the confines of his or her own limitations is the therapist I want for myself and my family.

Actually, therapists may care more about confidentiality than cops do. Sally Gross-Farina, a therapist, attorney, and former cop, wrote a funny and informative booklet for cops about counseling in which she warns cops not "to blame the therapist for our own loose tongues." If word is out that you and your spouse are seeing a marriage counselor, your kids are out of control, and you have financial troubles again, it may be because you or your mate told just one other cop who told just one other cop who told. . . .

SHOULD YOU OR SHOULDN'T YOU?

There is an endless number of reasons to start therapy. Some people start because their lives are unbearable, others because they are interested in personal growth. One thing is certain—you don't have to be nuts to be in therapy. It's enough to count yourself among the "worried well."

Common sense says you should go before you are sent or before your problems stack up so high you have a crisis on your hands. Multiple problems and crises make both your life and the shrink's job harder.

Consider this list of reasons for seeking therapy. If you have some of these concerns, it may be time for you to pick up the phone and make an appointment.

- Emotional pain
- Poor self-esteem
- Difficulties coping with everyday life
- High stress and/or stress-related medical problems such as headaches or hypertension
- Severe depression or the chronic blahs
- Anxieties, fears, phobias, and panic attacks
- Marital problems
- Sexual problems
- Relationship problems of all kinds
- Trouble with kids
- Trouble with parents
- Job problems; career concerns
- Grief that won't stop
- Addiction to drugs, alcohol, gambling, eating, or spending
- Big decisions to make
- Posttraumatic stress reactions
- Feeling stuck
- Nightmares; trouble sleeping

TROUBLED MARRIAGES

I really like the work of Dr. John Gottman, a marital therapist from Washington State. It's his contention that most couples wait six years to get help. By this time whatever's wrong in the relationship feels permanent and beyond fixing. Don't cheat yourselves by treating therapy as a last-ditch effort or a Code 3 call.

I've adapted and condensed some of Dr. Gottman's ideas to give you this list of warning signs. You can take his relationship quiz by visiting his website or reading one of his books (see the Resources for information).

Five Signs Your Relationship is in Trouble

1. The quality of your friendship is low. You no longer respect each other or enjoy each other's company. You know little about each other's preferences, aspirations, hopes, and gripes. You no longer do little things for each other or express interest

in each other's everyday lives. Friendship is so basic to a good marriage that, Dr. Gottman thinks, infidelity for some people represents a search for lost friendship.

2. There's more negative than positive in your relationship, in contrast to happy couples who have a 5:1 ratio of positive interactions. You are critical of each other and your life together much of the time. Pleasant memories don't override your bad ones.

3. Your discussions lead off with criticism and contempt. Communication is characterized by defensiveness and stonewalling. Either of you says whatever angry thing comes into your mind. Efforts to repair the damage fail or never happen. Once an argument starts, neither of you knows how to stop it. All couples get angry and fight; it's *how* you fight that counts.

4. You tolerate hurtful behavior in each other. Hurtful behavior exists along a continuum from lack of respect and consideration to outright abuse.

5. The man in the relationship won't accept influence from the woman. Women are used to accepting influence from men, Dr. Gottman says, but for a true partnership to exist, a man must do the same.

GETTING STARTED: WHERE TO LOOK AND HOW TO PAY

Cops and their families often have several options to choose from in terms of mental health professionals and mental health programs.

In-House Counseling Programs

Some departments offer *in-house* counseling programs where mental health professionals work for the department, full or part time. They may have offices in the department proper or in a separate facility. The in-house mental health provider can wear many hats: counselor, trainer, evaluator, crime scene consultant, or management advisor.

Many large agencies like the NYPD, LAPD, the FBI, and the Secret Service have in-house programs. They offer the advantage of on-the-spot availability and therapists who are familiar with the culture of the agency and the community. Likewise, the cops are familiar with the therapists and would confide in them more easily than they would confide in a stranger. The disadvantage of an in-house program is that many cops think there's a pipeline from the therapist's office to the chief. The fact that in-house therapists have many roles and are part of the organization may be a mixed blessing. You might see them in therapy one day and at a retirement dinner the next. Some people think that's great; others find it uncomfortable.

Out-House Counseling Programs

Out-house programs contract with independent counselors to provide a range of mental health services to employees. There is usually an in-house coordinator who manages the program—monitors quality control, utilization rates (which are usually reported by code, not name), cost containment, provider selection, and other administrative issues. The out-house providers may be located in one spot, such as a hospital or university counseling department, or the providers may work out of individual offices. The DEA, ATF, and many municipal police departments contract with off-site employee assistance programs.

The advantage of off-site programs is that they offer clearer boundaries between themselves and the police agency. Chances are you won't see your "shrink" at the annual picnic, and no one will see you walking into his or her office. The disadvantage is that the quality control of out-house programs varies: Some practitioners may know little about police culture, although that may not always be important to you, and they may also be inexperienced as therapists. Beyond that, some programs are so restrictive that you barely get started before your covered sessions are ended.

Medical Insurance

You and your family may be entitled to mental health benefits through your medical insurance, although there might be restrictions on the number of therapy sessions allowed and you may be required to pay some portion of the counselor's fee. Some insurance plans require that you get a referral from your physician and will pay only for certain services or providers: for example, outpatient, not inpatient treatment; psychologists, not social workers.

In any case, be prepared to pay something for therapy—either a copayment with your insurance carrier or the full fee to extend your allotted visits when they run out. Many therapists have sliding-scale fees and will negotiate with needy clients or those with financial emergencies. Therapy is expensive, but so are four-wheelers, jet skis, big houses, cars, and all the electronic toys many cops seem to be able to afford.

If you're on a restricted budget, check with your nearest family services agency, the Red Cross, or state or county associations for the various mental health disciplines, as well as the departments of social services or mental health. They will be able to refer you to low-cost counseling services or to therapists with sliding-scale fees. If you live near a university, see if they have a low-cost counseling clinic staffed by interns. Although interns are inexperienced, they do receive weekly supervision, so you might get the benefit of two mental health professionals for the price of one.

CHOOSING A THERAPIST

There are many different types of mental health practitioners and hundreds of different theoretical perspectives. Compassion, good listening skills, a supportive attitude, availability, integrity, and the fit between you and the therapist are more important than the letters after her name or his theoretical approach.

Psychiatrists (MDs) are medical doctors with specialized training in psychiatry. They can prescribe medication. Psychologists (PhD, PsyD, or EdD) have a doctorate plus 3,000 hours of supervised training. Clinical psychologists specialize in treating emotional or behavioral problems and psychological assessment. Social workers (MSW or LCSW) have a master's degree or a doctorate (DSW) plus supervised experience. Social workers are trained to consider social systems, as well as individual concerns. Master's-level therapists (MA and MS) have graduate degrees in psychology, marriage and family counseling, or a specialized field such as addiction counseling or grief counseling, plus supervised experience.

Finding the Treatment You Need

Psychotherapy doesn't come in a one-size-fits-all format. Just as you need to find a therapist with whom you have a good fit, the therapist needs to fit your treatment to your problem or refer you to someone who can.

There is a bewildering array of therapies available in some areas of the country and too few in others. People in California, where I live, can get analytic, autogenic, art, behavior modification, biofeedback, body, brief, Christian, crisis, client-centered, control-mastery, couple, cognitive, existential, family, feminist, Freudian, group, individual, neurolinguistic, primal-scream, psychodynamic, rational-emotive, reality, rebirthing, reincarnation, or shock therapy. And that's not the whole list.

In reality, therapists study various schools of thought and use a combination of strategies in their work. Still, some therapies are more effective than others in treating specific problems.

One of the best ways to find a therapist is to ask your friends. Get a name from someone who has been in therapy, feels good about the experience, and had positive results. You may run into problems if the therapist you want to see is not on the provider panel associated with your medical plan. Don't give up; see if you can nominate the therapist of your choice to your plan's panel.

Make certain the person you choose is a licensed mental health professional or a properly registered intern or psychology assistant. This is for your protection. Licensure and registration do not guarantee that a person will be helpful, but you will know that he or she has met the minimum requirements of training and supervision, carries malpractice insurance, and is bound by professional ethics. Beware—anyone can hang out a shingle and say he or she does counseling or psychotherapy. If you are uncertain, ask to see a license or check with the appropriate state licensing bureau. Certificates of competence or course completion are not equivalent to a state license.

It's okay to shop for a therapist. Ask questions about licensure, confidentiality, money, office policies, theoretical considerations—

whatever is on your mind. If the therapist doesn't want to discuss these issues with you or can't provide a satisfactory response, move on.

Use your gut instincts. You must feel comfortable with your therapist. Most programs will not penalize you for reasonable therapist shopping. On the other hand, give the therapist a chance to get to know you. If things aren't moving along by the third session, the chemistry probably isn't right. You can talk to your therapist about this and ask him or her for a referral. This is perfectly acceptable etiquette, and the therapist should be understanding and cooperative.

When you're looking for a therapist, ask about his or her strategies. Ask the therapist to give you a general assessment of your problems in lay terms and inquire if his or her approach is the best or only approach to treatment. It may be hard to think so rationally when you are in the midst of a crisis or are very emotional, but you can raise the question when things settle down.

Once therapy begins, don't expect miracles. Therapy has its ups and downs. Ask your therapist to estimate how long your treatment might take, but remember it's only an estimate. I was talking to Ernie the other day, who complained that six weeks of therapy hadn't cured him of 45 years of problems. Fifty minutes once a week is a drop in the bucket. Ernie should have been "working"—processing or observing what was happening to him between sessions, perhaps keeping notes or writing in a diary. He needed to tell his psychologist about what thoughts kept running through his head and what was turning up in his dreams. Instead, he sat back, waiting for the therapist to cure him. He wouldn't even tell the shrink how discouraged he was feeling about the therapy. I guess he expected the shrink to read his mind—something no mental health professional can do.

When you and your therapist agree that the time has come to stop, take time to close out your relationship with the therapist and review your work together. Wrapping things up can be a very rich installment in the therapy process. You have many options when you stop therapy. You can pick a date to stop or space out the time between sessions—from once a week to once a month. You can schedule "tune-ups" in advance or arrange for a telephone check-in. It's comforting to know that you can go back for a checkup now and then, before things build up.

Caveat Emptor

Most therapists are sincere, serious professionals with great integrity. The few bad apples tend to stand out. If your therapist frequently breaks appointments at the last minute with no reason, is a no-show, takes a lot of phone calls while talking to you, or falls asleep during your session, consider firing him or her and looking further. You can't get to first base in therapy if you can't get your therapist's attention.

Professional therapy *never* includes sex, flirting, improper touching, dating, or intimate socializing. If your therapist does any of these, you should end therapy. You also have the option of reporting this therapist to his or her licensing board.

Never agree to do anything in counseling that feels uncomfortable. If your therapist wants to record your sessions, videotape you, or have you talk to an empty chair, do it only if it is okay with you. If not, discuss your discomfort with the therapist. The bottom line is that you have a right to refuse any type of treatment or to end treatment without obligation or harassment. The department of consumer affairs in your state or county will provide you with a client bill of rights.

Most therapists avoid nonprofessional contacts with their clients. This may be hard if you live in a rural area where people run into each other all the time. It can complicate therapy, so if you can't avoid it, at least talk about it. Professional therapists will not barter services or goods for therapy. They should have a printed policy statement about their office practices and billing policies, and most will have some adjustable fee schedule for clients in need.

Buckle Your Seatbelt

There are many paradoxes in therapy—sometimes you have to lose control to get it back or feel bad in the service of feeling better. While the outcome of therapy can be enormously beneficial, as the *Consumer Reports* study shows, it may hurt along the way.

Be aware, too, that the outcomes of therapy are sometimes different from the ones you expected. You may get into therapy to figure out how to leave your spouse and wind up saving your marriage. Or you may bring your son in for treatment and discover that he is depressed because you and your mate are fighting all the time, and the way to help him is to help yourselves first.

Some change is unanticipated. What seems normal to you because you have lived with it for so long may change in the course of therapy—as it did for Stu, whose stomachaches were fueled by a tense and angry atmosphere at home. When things at home settled down, so did his stomach. Before therapy, he hadn't connected the two.

People enter therapy to change something. There are really only two things you can change, yourself and the furniture. You can modify other people's behavior through rewards and punishments or by changing the setting they are in, but you cannot really change their attitudes or personalities, unless they want to change.

To be successful, change must be achievable, manageable, and supportable. Often clients start therapy by looking for quick, drastic change. Jolie wanted *never* again to get angry at her kids, *always* to be understanding of her elderly mother, and *never* to be lazy, selfish, or cranky—despite being a single mom with a full-time, night-shift job. Her alternative plan was to change her kids and her mother. When she finished therapy, she wasn't the perfect woman she had hoped to be, but she had made one terrifically important change. She had learned to accept herself as she was, limitations and all. She was more self-disclosing and no longer put on a "tough cop" act while feeling scared and hollow inside. She had a sense of who she was, what she wanted to be, and a realistic self-appraisal. She still had a messy house and unruly kids, but she had learned some anger-management techniques and didn't blow up so much or so quickly anymore. She was still single, was overweight, and had continuing conflicts with her mother, but it was mild trouble now, and her mother's barbed criticisms never again hit home with the same power as before.

Jolie, Jenny, Duke, Lilly, Phil, Andy, Benny, and others in this book have profited from therapy. It may have been hard for them to get started, but they would now tell you that counseling or psychotherapy is an investment in yourself, your family, and your future. It takes guts to face problems and humility to ask for help, especially for cops. Seeking help when you need it is a sign of emotional health, not an indication that you are nuts or broken and need to be fixed. It means you are in pain and want to feel better. The individuals I worry about the most are the ones who are suffering in silence: who need assistance but can't bring themselves to get it until a possibly preventable crisis occurs.

PART III

SPECIAL FAMILIES, SPECIAL ISSUES

CHAPTER **12**

SWIMMING UPSTREAM

Special Challenges Facing Women, Minorities, Lesbians, and Gay Men in Law Enforcement

> It's like a hierarchy. The white males are on the top.
> Then the black males and any other minority males
> are the next best accepted. Then probably the white
> females. The black females are the least accepted.
> Except for the gay males—they're at the very bottom.
> —CONNIE FLETCHER, *Breaking and Entering*

A minority officer's experience is influenced by several factors:

- The climate of the organization where he or she works
- The degree of the organization's administrative and supervisory support
- The degree of the organization's commitment to fairness to all employees
- Community attitudes and politics
- Prevailing norms in society at large
- The number of other minority officers in the agency
- The officer's personality
- The officer's competence

Women make up nearly 12% of today's police force, a decline from recent years, and a fraction of the administrative ranks over sergeant. Ethnic minorities (African Americans, Hispanics, Asians, Pacific Islanders, Native Americans, and Alaska Natives) represent approximately 20%, and there are no available statistics on the percentage of gay and lesbian cops.

Being one of the few among many adds a unique element to the already significant strain of police work. Think of a time when you were one of the few because of age, occupation (yours or your mate's), religion, body size, politics, health status, social status, race, and so on. It makes no difference why you are in the numerical minority: You feel different, and people often treat you differently because of it.

When I am the only psychologist in a group of cops, I am almost always stereotyped as the bleeding heart liberal of the group—regardless of my actual views. People apologize for cursing in front of me, probably because of my age and gender, and they make funny remarks about my analyzing them on the sly. Some of these comments may be said with affection, but nonetheless, they serve to underscore how I am different from the group.

Numbers, of course, are not the whole story. Majority white male cops suffer considerable distress when they feel they and their families have been damaged by large social changes that are beyond their immediate control, such as affirmative action. Their distress is real and deserves attention. (See the Tips at the end of the chapter.)

Social change, even progressive change, creates painful dilemmas for everyone. Pat's story shows the problems of being a token and living in an unwelcome limelight. Pat was one of her department's first African American deputies. When a question came up about African Americans, coworkers would turn to Pat, as though she was the resident expert on what all black people, including crooks, thought and felt. This was amusing to her because she was raised in a suburban, middle-class household and had attended parochial school most of her life.

Shortly after she finished probation, Pat was asked to help the department in a stepped-up drive to recruit more ethnic minorities and more women. At first she was pleased and flattered at the assignment. She was sent to every job fair and high school career day in the state, but this caused her to miss a lot of patrol time.

The other cops were resentful and speculated that she wanted to be off the street because she couldn't take the heat.

Pat grew to be known as the administration's fair-haired girl—there were a lot of puns about that—and she began to lag further behind other cops as a competent field officer. She was being overexposed as a token at the same time that her real potential as a cop was being undermined and her career path delayed, perhaps even detoured toward a dead end.

Pat wisely sought out a former field training officer for advice. Juliet, who was now a sergeant, urged Pat to think about her career goals and begin to build a broad base of experience rather than get diverted into a specialty that served her agency's needs more than her own. This put Pat back on the right track in the nick of time.

WOMEN COPS: THE GENDER GAP

After her shooting, Lilly was astonished to find herself suddenly part of a fraternity she could never join before. Men who had shunned her for years as a colleague now patted her on the back for having killed someone. She was suspicious of their newfound camaraderie and sickened by the dues she had to pay to be considered a member of their club. An ardent feminist, she had worked hard to support and help other women. Now she had killed one and was being lauded for it.

A supervisor, who Lilly believed had once deliberately delayed other officers from coming to her aid while she was being pummeled by a suspect, sent her a congratulatory memo. A coworker, who had scathingly told her she would make a better social worker than a cop because she gave money to a homeless family, called to tell her what a good job she had done.

All this highlighted a profound difference between how Lilly and her male coworkers defined what it meant to be a good cop. Lilly's definition emphasized helping rather than controlling people. She regarded physical prowess, control and command actions, and officer safety as crucial skills cops need if they want to go home every night uninjured. But she didn't value these skills in the same way the men did. She felt most effective when she talked her way through a situation without the need for force. She thought many of the men relied too much on physical control and intimidation. She believed some overreacted to minor challenges and even looked for ways to exert their authority.

Coping with Harassment

There is less blatant harassment of women cops today than there was when they were first assigned to patrol duty. With few exceptions, from the mid-1800s on, women in law enforcement had been assigned stereotypically female tasks such as prison matrons and guardians of wayward women and children. Putting women on patrol was a radical move that threatened to destroy the very definition of what it meant to be a good cop, which was equated, and mostly still is, with being a "real man."

Over the years, women cops have suffered a rash of indignities. They've been fondled, insulted, ignored, and even raped. They've listened to lewd remarks and sexist jokes. They've found dead animals and used condoms in their mailboxes. They've been lied to, lied about, propositioned, and left without backup. They've been the subjects of gossip about their sex lives and their bodies. They've had no lockers or bathrooms of their own. They've been issued ill-fitting uniforms and bullet-proof vests designed for men. Their radio calls have been interrupted by clicking and scratching noises. They've been stuck in dead-end jobs and shut out of elite assignments like SWAT, canine, homicide, or motorcycle squads. When they've complained, they have risked retaliation and social ostracism—policing is not a job in which you can alienate your coworkers and then go to work every day and feel safe.

Things are better today, even though policing is still largely a man's world. And even though subtler forms of discrimination may have replaced or forced blatant harassment underground, the situation is much improved. Ask the Pengel sisters: Mindy is now deputy chief, her department's highest-ranked female. But when she was in the first academy class to have women, all the female rookies had to buck harassment, skepticism, and rejection every step of the way. When her two younger sisters, Miriam and Molly, joined the force years later, they had very different experiences.

For one thing, they joined a department that wanted them, and they had role models, like Mindy, to inspire them and smooth the way. They have the kind of acceptance and support that Mindy and others had been denied. As a result, they are able to focus their energies and enthusiasm on learning their jobs, not on proving themselves.

What Makes a Woman a Good Cop?

Women make a unique contribution to law enforcement, and a preponderance of studies show that they do the job with the same effectiveness as men—even when the task involves physical aggression, which is only about 10% of the time. The bulk of police work involves judgment, communication, investigation, negotiation, mediation, public relations, time management, report writing, and so on. The ideal cop is an androgynous combination of psychologist, minister, diplomat, politician, doctor, parent, historian, stunt-car driver, and sleuth.

The way women are culturally conditioned in our society prepares them to verbally defuse potentially explosive situations. They are more likely than men to talk someone down, rather than act aggressively when their authority is challenged. The Christopher Commission's investigation of the LAPD after the Rodney King incident found no women among the 120 cops with the most use-of-force reports.

In addition, women are at an advantage in undercover work because they are unexpected. They may also be more stress-resistant because they are apt to seek psychological help in a timely way, and they are less prone to alcoholism.

What challenges women specifically is not so much the physical rigor of the job—which challenges everyone, male and female officer alike, especially those who are out of shape or compromised by injuries—but a lingering mythology about what actually happens on patrol and the price women pay for being competent.

It is women's competence that is most threatening to those men whose self-esteem is based on being better and stronger than women; these men may privately welcome incompetent female cops because they fulfill the stereotype that women cannot do this work. It's a sad truth that there are such men around, though clearly not all male cops have so biased and condescending a point of view. There are enough, however, to impel one researcher, Joseph Balkin (1988), to bluntly claim that "the only trouble with women in policing is men in policing."

Damned if You Do/Damned if You Don't

Competent women are stuck between a rock and a hard place that men rarely if ever visit. It is hard for a woman to get due credit, unless she makes a mistake. When a women is promoted, the usual gossip is that she was promoted because of her gender, not on merit. A woman has to prove she is as good as any male officer, and she has to do this at every rank. Men need only to be as good as each other; they don't have to redefine themselves in the process.

On the other hand, when a woman shows she can be as aggressive, ambitious, powerful, proud, or tough as a man, she may get a reputation as castrating, pushy, or strident. She herself may feel defeminized, as if she has sacrificed part of who she really is and is acting tougher than she feels. She has to be masculine on the street but feminine in briefing; tough at work and nurturing at home—the demands change with dizzying speed and often inexplicable logic. It seems to make little difference whether the woman is lesbian or straight—she's still damned if she does and damned if she doesn't.

When Lulu was in training, her field training officer (FTO) gave her an unacceptable rating for failing to exert control over a loudmouthed prisoner who cursed at her as she filled out the booking sheet in a detention area. Her FTO said she could not allow prisoners to speak to her in a disrespectful manner. Lulu said that being called names was nothing to her and not worth escalating a bad situation or provoking a physical confrontation.

Her FTO accused her of being afraid to go hands-on with the prisoner and predicted she was too scared to be a deputy. Her other acceptable performance ratings were pushed to the background, and the cursing incident became symbolic of her overall performance. Subsequently, some training officers overprotected her because they were afraid she'd get hurt or might get them hurt. Others subjected her to higher standards of officer safety than the male rookies.

Lulu found herself in a Catch-22 predicament. She was increasingly reluctant to ask for backup in volatile circumstances because she felt it would reflect negatively on her ability to control the situation. At the same time, she was criticized for failing to ask for help. It was a great relief to her when she finally completed training and went out on her own. She had less scrutiny, fewer double messages, and more leeway to make decisions according to her own reading of a given situation. Because she was well trained, she completed her probationary year with no problems and went on to a successful career as a deputy sheriff.

On the Home Front

Many women complain that being a cop puts a damper on their social life. Some men are too intimidated to date or marry a female cop. Some men can't help but feel, and then can't deal with feeling, that the women in their lives are tougher and stronger or do more important work than they do. Others are cowed by women who are assertive and self-confident.

Some guys don't know how to respond to a woman who can be tough at work and then break into tears during a quarrel at home. They fail to recognize—perhaps because they don't have to do it themselves—how much gear shifting most women who work in male-dominated professions have to do to get by. No surprise, then, that the divorce rate among female cops is thought to be twice as high as for male cops.

Despite gains made by the women's movement, working women—cops included—often spend more hours on housework and childcare than men do. They feel more responsible for handling domestic tasks and for tending to relationship issues. Our culture teaches women that it is their responsibility to be available to listen to their mates' daily work hassles, even if they both do the same work, but not to insist or to expect the same level of support in return. Men seem to be able to get the support they want or need from their families, from their squads, from their supervisors, or by being rugged individualists, stoically bearing their problems alone—although this last way of coping creates more problems than it solves. Women cops rarely go it alone. They look mainly to their families for support and are often disappointed to find they provide more consolation than they receive.

Why Would a Woman Want to Be a Cop?

I asked a friend of mine who knows little about policing to read this section about women in law enforcement. She wrote the following note in a margin: "This is so depressing. Why would any woman want to be a cop?"

Women want to be cops for the same reason men do—they want secure, well-paying jobs that matter. Law enforcement offers more opportunities for variety, excitement, respect, and autonomy than do many jobs that are traditionally open to women. It pays better than the usual "women's work" and now offers possibilities for advancement. Shift work gives women opportunities for creative childcare arrangements, although there is a continuing need to develop better maternity and childcare policies.

Women entering law enforcement today still have the opportunity to be groundbreakers and influence law enforcement, both tactically and politically. They can be role models for young women. They can modify some of the rigid authoritarian practices that have contributed to negative public opinion and distrust of the police. They provide a needed service for women who are the victims of rape or domestic violence and find it hard to confide in male officers.

Culturally conditioned to be nurturers, women are uniquely suited to deal with quality-of-life issues and relationship building, which are the cornerstones of community policing—the wave of the future. Now, more than ever, opportunities exist for women to make significant contributions to law enforcement.

ETHNIC MINORITIES

Jorge, a Hispanic officer in training, was waiting at the door to my office. "I don't know if I can do this job, Doc," he said, "or even if I want to. I can't jam up every kid I see for being black or brown in public, which is what my training officer seems to want me to do. If I can't be a spirit-of-the-law cop instead of a letter-of-the-law cop, then maybe I don't belong in this business."

Jorge's training officer had ordered him to give curfew violation tickets to some Mexican kids who were sitting in a park, but he apparently ignored several groups of white kids who were doing exactly the same thing. Jorge thought this was unfair and punitive. At most, *all* the kids deserved a warning or a talking-to.

He'd sat in the same kind of park after curfew himself when he was a teenager. He remembered how he felt when he and his friends had gotten hassled by some officious white cops. He knew he didn't ever want to be that kind of cop.

When I suggested that Jorge talk this out with his FTO, he refused; he didn't want to risk getting a bad evaluation on his attitude. So he "stuffed" his feelings and decided that, if he was going to survive in this job, he would have to learn to pick his battles carefully and let a lot of things go by. The world was the way it was, and it wasn't his job to change it.

There are thousands of happy examples of friendship, loyalty, and genuine affection between cops of all races. But in the main, race relations between minority and majority police officers are as tenuous as they are for the rest of us. Many minority officers do not trust the majority officers to freely grant them the equal status prescribed by law, and many majority officers complain bitterly about being victims of reverse discrimination brought on by affirmative action. Some of these conflicts will be ironed out in the courts. But in the meanwhile, officers often work together under the shadow of contentious legal actions, court-ordered consent decrees, contested promotional processes, and the like.

Minority officers stand out from the group—in some departments more than others. They may feel scrutinized simply because they are more noticeable. Whether real or imagined, positive or negative, the attention that results from standing out can create undue strain for the person who is different.

Minority officers work in a culture that tends to stereotype minority races as criminal. The symbolic assailant in our collective cultural minds is a minority male, usually black. What are the psychological costs to a minority cop to be working side by side with a fellow officer who might believe that minorities are culturally, biologically, and inherently criminal? Who freely refers to minorities in demeaning slang and tells racist jokes? Who views a minority community primarily as a combat zone—a place to enhance arrest statistics and a prime training ground for rookies? What is the psychological damage of being undercover or responding to an off-duty incident only to be mistaken for the crook because a minority person with a gun is visualized as a crook, not a cop, in many cops' minds? What are the costs of being constantly reminded of your minority status in such demeaning ways?

Most minority officers want to be regarded not for their ethnicity but for their professionalism and their ability to be of service to anyone. Nonetheless, their ethnicity can be a valuable asset, although one they must use cautiously with minority suspects or coworkers for fear someone will accuse them of favoritism or expect special treatment.

Minority officers can make a big difference while working with people who are vulnerable to victimization and fearful of the police. Kheim, for example, is a traffic officer in a city with a large Vietnamese population. When he makes a traffic stop, he takes time to explain, in Vietnamese, how to fix the problem and reassures the driver that it is safe to deal directly with the authorities to pay tickets or warrants. He understands that many new immigrants are afraid of the police because they come from countries where the police are routinely corrupt and brutal. He suspects that when some of his colleagues make a traffic stop, they are really searching for serious criminal activity. If they don't find any, they quickly write a citation and leave. Sometimes the driver is too scared or confused to pay the ticket, which leads to more problems. Kheim believes his ability to relate to the driver and speak his or her language builds compliance with the law and more cooperation with the police when a serious crime does occur.

On occasion, Kheim's ancestry gets in his way. There are so many jokes about Asian drivers that when a non-Asian cop shows up at the scene of an accident involving Asians, Kheim sometimes feels embarrassed because the offenders are probably fulfilling that cop's expectations. He wants to lecture the offenders on their driving and shake them for perpetuating such foolish stereotypes. Then he wants to shake himself for feeling that way. Still, in all, he's glad that he is there to serve an underserved Vietnamese population and to bridge the gap between their community and the police. Under the present circumstances, he doubts that anyone other than a Vietnamese officer could establish that kind of rapport, particularly with newly immigrated residents.

The Juggling Act

Many minority officers feel they must juggle several allegiances, balance loyalties to different groups, and fill multiple roles that are often in conflict. Majority officers only rarely face such extremes.

Minority officers may belong to several unions or professional associations that are at odds with each other. They may serve civic or religious groups that are in conflict with the police. They may be viewed with suspicion by everyone.

All cops feel judged. They are perpetually scrutinized by the public, the courts, their superiors, and each other. But minority cops can feel judged by a set of complex standards. Sometimes it's hard for even the most sensitive majority officers to appreciate the subtle strains that minority officers and their families experience, especially those who feel marginalized at work and marginalized in their own communities.

Minority officers can serve as a bridge between their community and the police department. They can smooth the way for peaceful public demonstrations, gather information about community concerns, and act as a liaison between community activists and the police. These are high-risk ventures with potential for great gain to all involved, but they must be handled with sensitivity to the stress that goes along with managing multiple loyalties.

I ran into Jorge at a debriefing several years after our first meeting. He and some other cops had just arrested a Mexican man who fenced stolen goods out of a rented garage. There was an exchange of gunfire—the suspect's wife was injured, and his children were absolutely terrified. All of the officers, many of whom had little children, were chilled by the possibility that they could have injured or killed the children without even knowing they were there.

Some officers blamed the wife and called her a "piece of shit, just like her old man." Jorge knew differently and bristled at hearing her cheapened by the officers' ignorance about the culture. While he rarely spoke publicly about his personal life or his culture, he told me that traditional Mexican culture demands that women follow their men regardless of the path taken. He said this incident caused him to feel sorrowful for the times he had imposed strenuous demands on his wife and family.

Jorge wasn't excusing the fence for endangering his wife and children, but he could identify and empathize with the suspect's family in a way few others could. Instead of feeling isolated, Jorge felt proud of himself. He was pleased to be there to humanize the situation, to put a real face on a stereotype, to give voice to a voiceless woman. He was reassured that after all these years, he had not lost his identity as a Hispanic man or his compassion for people. His ethnicity distinguished him from others and deepened his insight into human behavior. He could and did do his job in the spirit of the law, the way he had hoped he could when he was a rookie.

GAY AND LESBIAN COPS

Tom was so good at being in the closet that when he finally came out, he had to convince people he was really gay. For years he had talked about nonexistent sexual exploits with women and laughed at jokes about "limp-wristed queers." There had been a lot of jokes, and the joke tellers came in all colors.

It was painful for Tom to stand by while his fellow cops mocked him without knowing it, minimized the epidemic of violence that plagued his gay friends, and treated gay crime victims with disdain or worse. He couldn't listen to his buddies talk about their fear of contracting AIDS without wondering if he would get life-saving help from them if they knew he was gay.

He had hung pictures of women in his locker, brought a woman friend to the Christmas party, and introduced his long-time lover, Ed, as a friend. He made up stories about what he did in his spare time and then grew anxious while trying to remember what he had said to whom. He was constantly on guard and on stage. He never invited people to the house he shared with Ed, and he dreaded the day that some cop he knew would see them shopping or eating out and put two and two together. It was hard for him to relax when off duty.

Ed, who was openly gay at his job, thought bigots should be in closets, not gays. He was proud of his relationship with Tom, proud of the home they shared, and wanted a more normal social life. There was tension between them because of this.

When Tom finally decided to come out of the closet, he did it in steps, starting with his partner, Ruben. It didn't go well at first. Ruben was angry about being "fooled" and hurt that Tom hadn't confided in him before. It took him longer to get over being lied to than it did for him to accept that Tom was gay. When he did, he jokingly threatened to recommend Tom for the next available undercover assignment because he was such a talented actor.

Tom was relieved. His worst fears were that Ruben wouldn't want to be his partner and would no longer be a reliable backup. After that, Tom took things slowly and did what came naturally to others but was daring for him. He put Ed's picture on his locker and talked about what they did over the weekend. He brought Ed to social events and invited people over to dinner. It was a great relief to him to be out and not as big a deal as he had thought. There were some remarks made and some obscene phone messages on his voice mail, but overall, most people were supportive or neutral.

Two things helped Tom make his decision to come forward. He had always been well liked, competent, confident, and hard-working, and he correctly believed that people would continue to accept him for those attributes. He also had faith that his department supported his rights and that any harassment he suffered for being gay would cost the offender his or her job. He boosted his own courage with the thought that he would not just make things easier for himself but that he could dispel a few stereotypes and pave the way for other closeted gay cops.

Gay cops have a staggering number of virulent stereotypes to overcome. Many police officers see themselves as protecting the moral order of society, and to some cops the idea of a homosexual cop is immoral.

As with women, gay men are presumed by some to lack such "manly" attributes as courage, bravery, and loyalty. And, like women, when they demonstrate courage and competence, they threaten the cherished notion that only "manly" men can do police work.

Curiously enough, lesbian women have told me that things are easier for them. They are less threatening to the status quo than gay men—some straight guys who are repelled by gay men are titillated by the thought of lesbian sex—and more often stigmatized for their gender than their sexual orientation.

Gays and lesbians don't choose their sexual orientation; they are probably born with it. But they can choose to be public or private about it because it is not overtly obvious in the way race or gender is. This is a highly individual decision, with immense consequences and legal overtones. Homosexuals are not a protected class and can be fired in some states simply because they are gay, even if they never have sex. Other states have penal statutes regarding specific sexual acts. These statutes are irregularly enforced, but they serve as a deterrent for openly declaring one's homosexuality.

Despite these obstacles, studies show that most, but not all, openly gay cops think the rewards of coming out far outweigh the costs, although the costs can be high. This was Betty's experience. She had been a cop for several years when she came out publicly in an interview with a local gay newspaper. She was totally unprepared for what was to follow—both the bad and the good. She and her family received anonymous hate mail and death threats at their homes and their jobs. Betty never knew when she was sitting next to the person who had just sent her a vile message. Her car was vandalized in the police parking garage, and she was the subject of grotesque gossip.

But Betty also received an unexpected show of support from the community at large and from many in the gay community. Like Tom, she was regarded as a good role model and a strong counterbalance to the prevalent stereotypes about gays. She was surprised at the number of straight parents of gay children who praised her for being someone their kids could look up to.

She grew closer to many people she worked with and realized with surprise that many of her coworkers had wondered all along if she was gay or straight but were reluctant to ask. Now that she was out and the barriers were down, she found her relationships with coworkers were more relaxed because no one was tiptoeing around. In fact, her cop acquaintances weren't as shocked at her being a lesbian as her gay friends were at her being a cop.

Tips for Helping the Minority Cop

- Encourage connecting with mentors, role models, or peers—people who can provide guidance, sponsorship, and information. Having informal networks is how people compensate for being left out of the formal ones.
- Encourage getting all the training and experience needed to build street skills since your loved one will be judged first and forever by his or her field experience. It is a peculiarity of the culture that an excellent administrator will be demeaned for having been a lousy street cop years ago.
- Encourage joining an association of other minority cops (see the Resources section). Minority cops are often wary of joining groups for fear of being seen as seeking special treatment at the same time they are insisting on parity. But the support and practical assistance these associations offer can balance the potentially negative consequence of joining them.
- Have a support system of your own. You, too, may be a target of the same bias that affects your cop. You may need someone to fortify you while you buoy up your mate. Don't forget the diverse support networks in your community or at your church.
- If your loved one is a victim of harassment or discrimination, encourage him or her to get mental health counseling or peer support. Victims of harassment, especially if they are unsupported by their agencies, need help to manage depression or anxiety.
- Be a confidence builder, problem solver, and good listener. Argue with catastrophic thinking. Cops who have a "deal with it" attitude and the confidence to challenge sexist, racist, and homophobic attitudes seem to fare better than those who feel helpless or ashamed.
- Provide objective feedback. Women are culturally conditioned

(cont.)

(continued from previous page)

to blame themselves for their misfortunes and to turn their anger inward. Men may turn their anger onto others. Help your cop sort through difficult times by providing calm, accurate feedback. Encourage fixing the problem, not the blame.

- If you know a female officer who is trying to be one of the boys, remind her that although she may need to add some "male" skills to her tool kit, she does not have to relinquish or exchange who she is to do so.

- Studies show that homosexual officers seem to fare better in larger, urban agencies, where there are more openly gay officers. The same may be true for women and ethnic minorities. The wise applicant will check out a prospective agency's antidiscrimination policies and find out if they are enforced.

- Never push your cop to come out, speak up, file a lawsuit, start a grievance, and so on. These are tough decisions, and the person who must live with the consequences is in the best position to decide how to proceed.

- Beware of rigid sex roles. Talk about the division of labor in your household and hold to a reasonable standard of order and cleanliness—not the spit-and-polish standards required at work.

- Fight stereotypes. Female officers should not let anyone assume that they don't want to be considered for certain jobs—midnights or narcotics—because they are women, wives, or mothers. Remind everyone that a female cop is still a cop.

- Now that men and women are working side by side in law enforcement, there is room for jealousy, which is an unbearable and destructive emotion. Try to get to know your mate's coworkers as people. Invite them to get to know you. Concentrate on the strengths and weaknesses of your own relationship before assigning the source of the trouble to someone else.

- Assert your right not to be insulted or drawn into offending others. Don't be discounted by people who tell you that you are too sensitive or you don't understand the hard-hitting cop humor.

(cont.)

(continued from previous page)

- Don't forget your history. Many senior cops see their younger colleagues as naive or complacent about the status of women or minorities in police work. It is not necessary to be paranoid, just to be informed and aware.
- Minority officers often have opportunities to get financially lucrative undercover assignments by working narcotics or vice in a minority neighborhood. If they put money in front of advancement, they may stay so long in these assignments that they forfeit any opportunity to advance beyond the rank of officer. Encourage your officer to take a long-range view of his or her career. Make every effort to live within your means and not depend on the artificially inflated income produced by massive overtime.

Tips for Helping the Majority Male Cop

- Remind your cop that it is normal to experience anger and frustration when he thinks he is being punished for long-standing, major social problems he didn't create.
- Lost opportunities for majority officers are bound to happen as our society struggles and experiments with multiculturalism and diversity. It helps to be prepared for the possibility that your cop's career may be affected.
- Encourage your cop to talk out his strong feelings with others, peers or professionals, rather than bottling them up, turning them on himself, or blaming others.
- Try to separate what you can control from what you can't.
- Don't be quick to assume that your cop's majority status is what keeps him from certain opportunities. You and he may overlook something that can be changed to his advantage.
- Use an experience of being "shut out" to understand how much damage discrimination inflicts on everyone.
- Encourage your cop not to put all his eggs in the "cop" basket. Urge him to find more ways than work to feel valued.

CHAPTER 13

COP COUPLES

Our very first intimate night together, I sat down on
the bed and took off my gun and badge. . . .
I looked over the bed and she's doing the same thing.
That was a little bit of a shock.
—OFFICER VINCE ROGERS,
Stress in the Police Family

Being a cop couple has lots of advantages. When it comes to
work, cops understand each other without having to go into long
explanations or answer a lot of questions. They listen without
overreacting because they've probably been through a similar
event. They know the same people. They've had the same training. They share a sense of gallows humor that would repel most
civilians. They benefit from each others' experience. In times of
stress, they can support each other with feedback, counsel, and
perspective. They can help each other in practical ways—coaching
for interviews, studying together for promotional tests, and planning for career decisions. They make good money. They are good
problem solvers. Those with kids can arrange shift work to their
benefit so that they each have some time to themselves, and the
children have one parent at home nearly all the time.

There are also a lot of dilemmas facing cop couples, though
perhaps no more than any other dual career pair. They see each
other too little. They talk about nothing else but work. They have
a double dose of job stress. They feel competitive. They worry
about not spending enough time with their kids. They have far
too much to do and too little time to do it in.

MEL AND JOANNE: STEADY PARTNERS

Mel and Joanne are a good example of the benefits of being a cop couple and the wisdom of making the job work for the family, not the other way around. They have been married for 15 years and have three young children. They work as lieutenants in the same large, urban agency. Both are self-confident, ambitious, organized, and devoted to their family.

Mel and Joanne met in the police academy. They grew up in the city where they work and have lots of childhood friends and family around. After they married, they made a conscious choice not to live where they worked and moved to a nearby suburb. They spend a lot of time socializing with the parents of their children's friends. Their combined salaries make them financially comfortable and allow them to indulge their mutual passion for sailing.

When they first married, they made some decisions that have held up well over time. They decided never to work the same beat. For one thing, they wondered if they could remain objective if either was verbally challenged or physically assaulted in front of the other, something that was bound to happen. After they had children, they were especially conscious of safety issues and had to consider the unlikely possibility that they could both be injured at the same time or their children could be left without parents.

They also decided that while they would try to balance work and family responsibilities, they would put their family first rather than volunteer for various committees or attend department-sponsored social activities in their off-duty hours. They have paid a price for that decision—neither has a select assignment that puts him or her in line for further promotion. They consider it a small price for family unity.

Working in a Fishbowl

Their professional lives have not been easy. They work in a fishbowl: Everyone knows their business—how much money they make, when they go on vacation, and when one is promoted and the other is not. If they come to work in different cars, people ask if they are separated. If Joanne goes out to lunch with a male coworker, it's assumed she's having an affair. They are the subjects of rumors, gossip, envy, and jealousy. Mel is constantly ribbed about Joanne's rank—his buddies want to know who wears the pants at home? Does she wear her bars in bed? Social situations can be especially awkward. Some cops don't know if they should treat Joanne as Mel's wife or as a superior officer. Civilian wives keep their distance. Joanne thinks she gets twice the usual animosity aimed at women in law enforcement.

Mel is emotionally secure, which is a good thing since Joanne was promoted before he was. He derives his security from his family, not his job, and has always maintained an optimistic outlook about his future, separate from his achievements at work. If he has felt competitive, it has been with himself, not Joanne. This has helped him deflect the sarcastic remarks about being "Mr. Mom" or not earning enough money to support the family by himself.

Spillover

At times, the job has spilled over into their family life, contaminating the tranquility of their home. Joanne has been affected by her work on child abuse cases. She just can't shake the memories of small children with terrible physical and mental injuries. She might be bathing her son and suddenly flash back to a little boy whose mother had forced him to sit in scalding water. Once, her daughter complained of a pain between her legs and Joanne panicked, thinking her daughter had been sexually abused. She had to calm herself down before she could ask questions and determine that her daughter had hurt herself on the monkey bars at school.

Joanne has told Mel about her child abuse cases, and talking has helped put things in perspective. But she has been careful to protect him from the specific details of what she has seen because she doesn't want to "pollute" his mind with disturbing images. This is a hard call to make. As cops, you see so many distressing things. It really helps to talk and not bottle stuff up. At the same time, you want your relationship to be a port in the storm, a place to hide out from work and from the world. Sometimes it's hard to know when to talk and when to shield your mate from disturbing details. On the other hand, because you do see so much despair, random violence, and loss, you can more deeply appreciate each other and what you have together. You know better than most couples not to take things or each other for granted.

Managing Time

Mel and Joanne are very organized. They have to be because scheduling is a big problem. They have a family calendar in the kitchen, and *everything* is written down in advance: vacations, school holidays, training obligations, special school activities, family visits, household chores, medical appointments, and so on. Fortunately, they both get their schedules a year in advance, so except for occasional emergencies, they can and do make plans they stick to. Shift work has allowed Mel to be much more involved with his kids than his father was with him. On the downside, working midnights for years caused Mel some medical problems that were related to sleep deprivation.

Both Mel and Joanne are family-friendly managers. They try to accommodate the parents on their shifts. By contrast, they occasionally run afoul of the few remaining old-guard administrators when one of them needs to adjust his or her hours or take time off because the other is on special assignment.

Not every cop couple is as fortunate or as well grounded as Mel and Joanne, and not every cop couple would make the same choices. But Mel and Joanne are a good example of what it takes for two cops to sustain a relationship.

- Loyalty to each other and the family
- Satisfying work
- A diversified social network and support system to supplement the family
- A range of interests and recreational activities outside of policework
- Self-esteem
- Willingness to give and receive support
- The ability to have fun
- Patience to endure the hard times

- Optimism to know that bad times won't last forever
- Good coping skills—problem solving, time management, and planning for the future
- Good health and high energy

BONNIE AND MARK: ON A ROLLER COASTER

Bonnie and Mark's life has been quite different from Mel and Joanne's. Today, they are at a crossroad in their marriage, trying to stay positive in light of an uncertain future.

Working in a Fishbowl

Bonnie and Mark were partners long before they became lovers. They were an odd couple—she was one of the first women in the department, and he was one of the first Asians. Rumors about their relationship began before they became romantically involved. Everyone just assumed they were sleeping together because what other reason would a guy have for partnering up with a woman? The teasing never let up. If they didn't answer the radio immediately, they got ribbed about making love in the patrol car.

Bonnie fought to get some attention as a cop, not as a woman. Mark fought to keep their privacy. Neither one was very successful. The pressure they experienced pushed them together— a sort of us-versus-them reaction—and spurred them to keep working as partners after they became romantically involved. This was a decision they later regretted.

Spillover

At first they liked working together and relished having the same shifts and days off. They remember this as the best of times: Love was new; the job was fresh; they were surrounded by novelty and excitement. In the beginning they were able to separate their personal and professional lives. They would put quarrels behind them when they came to work and leave work behind when they went off their shift.

Eventually it grew harder to maintain the boundaries, and difficulties cropped up in unanticipated ways. Bonnie was certain of Mark's fidelity, so she was surprised to catch herself feeling jealous of other women. When they made traffic stops, she hated watching women drivers primp in their rear-view mirrors in hopes of impressing Mark and wheedling themselves out of a ticket. She always insisted, with perverse pleasure, that she be the one to get out of their patrol car and issue the citation. She noticed her manner was less than courteous.

One day Mark hit someone who called Bonnie a bitch and spat at her. It wasn't because he thought she couldn't defend herself: Mark always thought Bonnie was a competent street cop. But he was filled with rage and confused for the moment by juggling so many roles—cop, partner, and lover—all at the same time. Bonnie, in turn, was angry at his inappropriate gallantry. They didn't talk on the way home or all the next day. The atmosphere in their patrol car was icy.

When you talk to Bonnie and Mark now, they'll tell you flat out that they had let the job consume them and that that was a big mistake. They had few friends outside of the department and virtually no other interests. Police work was literally all they had to talk about.

Double Crisis

On one occasion, Mark and Bonnie got into a huge brawl during a bar check. Mark was badly hurt. It would have bothered Bonnie greatly to have any partner of hers injured in the line of duty, but she took this incident especially hard because she felt she should have shot the thug who stomped Mark and thus prevented the whole thing. Mark thought she was right to follow her instincts; after all, she could have shot *him* by mistake. But Bonnie couldn't shake off the self-doubt. The mood at home was grim. He was hurt and on disability leave; she was terribly depressed.

Mark received some discipline for the bar fight, adding insult to injury as far as he and Bonnie were concerned. Bonnie actually took the reprimand harder than he did. He was glad for her support and empathy and the fact that they interpreted the event in the same way—this was a political maneuver, and he was being used to set an example. But in the long run, all they did was depress each other more. They were both in a funk: Neither one could raise the other's spirits.

Mark was lonely and jealous because Bonnie was out working while he was laid up at home. He started to drink. Bonnie would come home from work and find him stone drunk in front of the TV set, watching some cop show. She was desperate for help but too afraid to tell anyone at the department because she didn't want to get him in any more trouble. Months later, after Mark returned to work, Bonnie approached Mark's supervisor and asked for help. He offered her no advice except to suggest that she should "babysit" Mark and make sure he didn't drink on the job.

Soon, they began fighting in earnest over Mark's drinking. They were acting like two cops in battle mode. He raised his hand to her, and she put him in an arm lock. She went for her baton, and he threw her down like a prisoner. They separated for a short while, and they then switched partners during the separation. It was extremely hard on both of them to see each other at briefing or roll up on each other's calls.

Mark developed a bleeding ulcer and was carted off to the hospital in an ambulance. This incident motivated him to get into a treatment program for his drinking, and he and Bonnie reconciled. Shortly after that, Bonnie blew out her knee chasing a suspect. When she was able to return to work, she decided she'd had enough of patrol duty and transferred to the crime prevention bureau.

Mark has done well since treatment. He is physically healthy and in a good place emotionally. But times are rough for Bonnie— she's lost both her partner and her job. She likes crime prevention, but she's envious when she listens to Mark's war stories about the fun and excitement he has with his new partner. She's getting bored doing commercial inspections and talking to neighborhood watch groups. There's value in what she does, but she misses the adrenalin rush from being on the street.

Now that Bonnie and Mark no longer work together, they wonder what they have in common. Bonnie has enrolled in real estate school because she thinks she may not last in this job until retirement. She just turned 42 and is feeling her age. Her doctor told her if she hurts her knee again she will be permanently disabled. Mark is taking courses in Chinese cooking and woodcrafting. He goes to AA meetings and knows that he has to find interests outside of work to remain sober. Both of them understand that they have to break free from the work cocoon they have inhabited for most of their marriage if they are to stay together.

Bonnie and Mark have had a tough time—some of it of their own doing and some just bad luck. They made choices that they thought were right but that didn't serve them well over the long haul. They walked into almost every pitfall facing cop couples.

- They were addicted to work.
- They treated their relationship as a refuge and had too few outside interests or friends.
- They depended on each other for so much that they literally suffocated one another.
- They had poor communications skills—they didn't know how to fight well, so they used silence and withdrawal instead of dealing with the issues directly. On the other hand, they sometimes fought just to get some distance from each other and the emotional intensity at home. Eventually, they resorted to physical force.
- They were too proud and too fearful to get help when they most needed it.
- They did not think ahead and were unprepared for the possibility that injuries would force one of them to retire prematurely.
- Their personal life was contaminated by too much job-related negativity. They didn't have enough positive activities in their lives to offset it.

KRISTEN AND GARY: GROWING APART AND STAYING TOGETHER

Mel and Joanne's and Bonnie and Mark's lives together have had a certain symmetry. Mel and Joanne have followed parallel paths. Bonnie and Mark have traveled a more tumultuous route, but they have done so together, until Bonnie's recent injury. In contrast, Kristen and Gary have led asymmetrical lives—she has been successful and happy in her work, and he has not. This is a difficult situation for any dual-career couple, requiring each to make tremendous accommodations for the other without sacrificing individual goals. It also forces the couple to resist being pressured by prevailing social norms that imply something is awry when a wife is more successful than her husband.

Kristen and Gary have been married 18 years and have two children, one in high school and one in college. Gary has a grown son from a previous marriage. They were both rookies in training when they met at an interdepartmental charity softball tournament. Gary worked for a large municipal agency, and Kristen worked for the state police.

Off to a Good Start

Life couldn't have been more exciting. They were intensely attracted to each other and initially filled with enthusiasm over their new careers. Being a cop was like nothing either had done before. Their shared passions overshadowed their considerable differences. Gary had grown up in a large, traditional family: His father had worked, and his mother had managed things at home. His life was secure and predictable, and he had wanted for nothing. His greatest pleasures and greatest successes came from his athletic abilities.

Kristen had grown up in a military family. She rarely saw her father, who was away most of the time. Her family had moved more than a dozen times before she started junior high school. Her parents' marriage was deeply disappointing to both of them and ended in divorce when Kristen was in the eighth grade. Her mother's life was very hard after that. As a consequence, Kristen made up her mind that she would never depend on a man for survival. She set herself a series of goals to achieve this independent status. Her first goal was to be the first in her family to get a college degree, which she did before entering the academy.

Kristen was initially very frustrated with law enforcement. She was used to being successful and popular. She had never before encountered overt sexism, and she was dumbfounded by the hostility she received simply because she was a woman. Gary was a major help to her. He encouraged her to stick with it when she was ready to give up. He helped her to deal with narrow-minded coworkers and to understand the male culture. She credits his early encouragement with her later success.

Gary, on the other hand, took to law enforcement like a duck to water. He loved the thrills and excitement and put in for every high-risk specialty assignment he could find: SWAT, motorcycles, the drug task force, and so on. But six years later, he was starting to feel burned out. He thought about putting in for a promotion, but he was ambivalent about missing the street work. He had never gone to college, something his department required for promotion, and at age 36, he was older than many of his superior officers.

Once she had completed training, Kristen was deployed to a command post that was very supportive of women. She received some plum assignments and was recognized for her contributions and talents. She was a natural-born manager; she had grown up managing her sisters and brothers. And she was a compulsive planner, which is an asset for administrators who need to think ahead in 5- and 10-year increments.

Growing Apart

Their common ground started to fall away. Gary, like many cops, was a spur-of-the-moment guy who relished the hands-on aspect of law enforcement. He had no interest in budgets or long-range strategic planning. Kristen had no interest in SWAT. He was still on patrol, while she was rapidly moving from assignment to assignment and promotion to promotion. He had little in common with her coworkers and friends; she had little in common with his.

Unlike in the early days of their relationship, they were no longer able to impress the other with their respective accomplishments at work. Dinner-table conversations were strained. Gary was frustrated by his department and resentful of several marginally qualified females whom he suspected got special privileges simply because they were women. When he tried to talk about his frustrations, Kristen got defensive and accused him of thinking she, too, was successful merely because she was a woman. It became a subject they couldn't discuss because they were each too emotionally involved.

Having Kids

They both agree on one thing: Having children made things worse. Their first child didn't totally disrupt their life: They could still hike and go out to dinner. But they felt pressured to have a second child as soon as possible before Kristen got much older. Having two infants in diapers was considerably harder to manage and had a much greater impact on their relationship.

Gary felt as though he had lost his last major connection to Kristen—their shared interest in sports. They went from being lovers to friends to roommates. The only common ground they now had was the children and perpetual remodeling of their house. Gary felt that the only reason Kristen and the kids needed him was to pound nails and fix leaks. He resented sharing Kristen with her job—which as a manager required her to put in long hours—and resented sharing her with the kids. He handled his resentment by withdrawing into himself. The more he withdrew, the more she turned to the kids.

Kristen was overwhelmed with childcare responsibilities. She was angry with Gary for expecting her to take care of him, as well as the children. He admired and supported her successes at work, but she felt as though he also expected her to take care of most of the household chores—which was what he was used to when he grew up.

Gary was at a dead end. He was losing his physical stamina and accumulating injuries. He felt all he had to show for his years of experience was a better choice of shift. He had outgrown the things that had once made his job worthwhile and stimulating.

Kristen tried to encourage him to go back to school. She helped him study for promotional exams. But the more she helped, the more he resented her. He accused her of trying to manage him the way she managed people at work. In retrospect, she wishes she had listened more and offered less advice. But she was frightened by how depressed and withdrawn he had become, and her automatic take-charge response was to push harder.

It was the worst of times; they hardly spoke unless it was about the kids. Kristen felt uncomfortable talking about her successes; Gary felt humiliated talking about his failures. Consciously, he wanted her to succeed; unconsciously, he sabotaged her efforts by "forgetting" he was supposed to watch the kids while she had an important public appearance or by keeping her up all night talking before a critical interview.

Taking a Risk

The break came when Gary's brother Chuck asked Gary to help out in his property management firm. Chuck's partner had been killed in an automobile accident, and Chuck couldn't handle the business alone. Kristen encouraged Gary to take it. She assured him that her salary alone could see them through if it didn't work out. She tried to convince him that he was a really capable person who had stayed too long in the wrong profession. She truly believed he would be much better off as his own boss.

Leaving law enforcement helped their situation a lot. Gary no longer felt like an underachiever compared to Kristen. He was intellectually stimulated by this new set of challenges and motivated to return to school for his degree in business accounting. That felt like an enormous accomplishment, and for the first time in a long while, he began to feel as though he had some value and was interesting to Kristen again because he now had some expertise in an area she knew little about. Their kids were older, and they now had more free time as a couple. Gary had more things to contribute to the kids—coaching their soccer teams and taking them camping.

An Uncertain Future

Kristen and Gary are still tentatively feeling their way forward. They are sorry Gary didn't take a risk and leave law enforcement years ago. On the other hand, changing careers hasn't totally erased the consequences of years of doubt, discouragement, and emotional distance. On occasion Gary frets that what he now does for a living doesn't have enough social meaning and may not sustain his interest. Kristen worries that her continuing successes obscure his accomplishments and that she asks for more support from him and the family than she gives in return. He worries that he is not sufficiently supportive of her. The male administrators he knows all seem to have wives who run their homes and accompany them to endless social functions and public appearances, seemingly without complaint. Gary can't and won't do this very often—he is socially introverted and feels uncomfortable running into his former bosses.

Neither knows what the future holds. Gary's business is doing so well that he and his brother are thinking of branching out to other locations. He shudders at the thought of asking Kristen to give up her job and move. Kristen, on the other hand, has realistically set her sights on positions of increasing responsibility and visibility. Every one of them would require her to relocate the family. She is terrified of asking Gary to pull up stakes for her sake just when he seems settled and happy.

Gary's and Kristen's life together illustrates the fortitude and persistence required of dual-career couples in order to be successful as partners, parents, and professionals. There were many times when each would have given up—Kristen on her career and Gary on himself and the marriage—were it not for each other's encouragement. They helped each other avoid handling anxiety by making impulsive decisions.

For the most part, they were able to assume responsibility for their own problems rather than point fingers at each other. Gary was usually able to be respectful and admiring of Kristen's accomplishments, even when he was feeling terrible about himself. Kristen could almost always regard Gary as a worthwhile person. He did not blame his failure to be promoted on her, and she did not claim her achievements were made in spite of him.

Although they did a lot of distancing from each other, they were mostly able to set their own problems aside and cooperate as parents. As a consequence, they have good relationships with their kids, and the kids are well adjusted and content.

They now take a long-range view of their marriage—seeing it as a work in progress, with some years better than others. They do not harbor resentment over past problems but seem to be able to again enjoy each other's company.

Tips for Cop Couples

- Plan for the future: It takes a lot of discussion and careful planning to balance your career goals with your family goals. Be realistic, especially if you are a woman, about how children will change your lives. Figure out what childcare resources will be available to you. Discuss in advance how you will share your domestic responsibilities.

- Attend a family orientation or couple training class at your academy or agency. Don't imagine you know it all or that as a cop couple you will be out of place with other couples in which one spouse is a civilian. The basics of a successful relationship are the same regardless of what either spouse does for a living.

- Make an emergency childcare plan for your family. In case of a big incident—an earthquake, a riot, a hostage situation—both of you may be working overtime. Join or form a babysitting cooperative and babysit for friends and neighbors whenever possible; then you can call in your IOUs in an emergency. Except for emergencies, don't use childcare as an excuse not to do something. People may think you are not serious about your career or that you expect preferential treatment.

- Don't let others assume that you can't handle competing against each other or that the more important opportunities should automatically go to the male partner first. You will need to make adjustments to help each other's career, but if either of you sacrifices too much for the other, you may lose too much of yourself and the attributes that attracted you to each other in the first place.

- Diversify your interests: Having a variety of activities, hobbies, or subjects that intrigue you makes you more intriguing to each other. Shop talk gets boring faster than you think. Relying on your mate as your only source of emotional stimulation puts too much pressure on the relationship. Having interests of your own is a great solace when your mate is working or you are feeling temporarily last in line for his or her attention.

(cont.)

(continued from previous page)

- Take time out to do things completely unrelated to police work or cops. It may be fun to go to the Police Olympics every now and then, but you will talk shop, as well as sports. Don't make that your only vacation. Make a real effort to expose your kids to more of the world than you see in your jobs. Couples who engage in physical activity together seem to fare better than those who don't.

- Develop support systems outside of your family. You may need them if you are both on a downswing or if you are concerned that sharing something with your spouse will hurt him or her more than it helps you to talk. Because you love someone doesn't mean you automatically understand that person or that he or she always knows how best to support you. In the unlikely event that you are both involved in the same critical incident, you may each need more than you have to give.

- Structure your time so that you have some off-duty time together, some with your kids and some by yourself. Both partners have to negotiate this to meet their own needs.

- Try to balance work and home life. Set your priorities and be flexible enough to revise them as you go along because things change. Be as clear as you can about defining what you consider to be a good balance. Negotiate your differences rather than compromising so much that neither of you feels as if you are getting what you need. Set goals for yourself as a couple, as a family, and as individuals.

- Don't let anyone but yourself design your career around your children. Some departments make assumptions that women won't want tough assignments after they become mothers. You may have needed a desk job when you were pregnant, but if you allow yourself to get stuck there while your husband works more meaningful or exciting assignments, it can lead to jealousy and resentment. It can detour your career, as well as your marriage.

- Cops are by training critical and analytical. What may seem to be a helpful comment made out of genuine concern for your loved one's safety can be taken as a hurtful put-down.

(cont.)

(continued from previous page)

Giving and receiving feedback is negotiable. Always ask your mate *if* he or she wants your advice or feedback. It is not your job to train your mate. Sometimes family members are just too invested in each other to be helpful, no matter how much both of them would like it to be otherwise.

- Cops are by nature competitive, which can be a very positive trait but can also lead to anger and hurt. You can avoid direct competition by specializing in different aspects of policing or working in different departments or agencies.

- There's enough anecdotal evidence to suggest that cop couples have a higher-than-average incidence of domestic violence in their families. The physical control you must exert on the street is never appropriate at home. Seek help at the first sign that either you or your mate is behaving in a physically, emotionally, or verbally abusive manner toward each other or toward your kids. Review Chapter 9 and see the Resources for more information on domestic abuse.

PART **IV**

SUMMING UP

CHAPTER 14

SUCCESS STORIES

> "I'll get over this," she said. "I've always been good at it. Getting over things."
>
> "I know," he said. "I know some of the things you've managed to get over."
>
> "Oh, my boy, you couldn't even guess."
>
> —E. ANNIE PROULX, *The Shipping News*

BENNY: BACK ON TRACK

I ran into Benny the other day by accident. He was the officer in Chapter 4 who had been charged with excessive force and despaired of ever recovering sufficiently from that incident and its aftermath to be able to do his job with confidence and satisfaction. Benny looked wonderful—fit, healthy, and relaxed.

"Things are going great," he told me. "I'm a different man—more easygoing, more confident—not much gets me riled up anymore. You're not going to believe this, Doc," he said, and then he told me about a barking-dog call he recently handled. It was the kind of call that he would previously have regarded with impatience and irritation because it wasn't "real" police work. It took a lot of time and follow up, but he seemed genuinely pleased to have been of service to an elderly couple, who later wrote him a letter of commendation.

Benny looked and felt secure because his future as a cop was once again assured. He appears to have enough control over himself to no longer worry about blowing up and getting in trouble. He and the chief he once mistrusted have established a decent working relationship. His current successes are largely due to his own efforts, but his own efforts would not have been sufficient had everyone not agreed on the ultimate outcome—they wanted Benny to be rehabilitated and get back to work.

On the home front, Benny's marriage to Carole seems to have weathered those horrible months with little permanent damage, and they have finally started the family they have wanted for so long.

It was a treat for me to hear about Benny's successes. When we began working together, I was more pessimistic than optimistic about his future as a cop. Fortunately, I was wrong. Instead, Benny was able to snatch his career back from the brink of disaster through a combination of his own endeavors and his chief's willingness to give him a fair chance. He wins, his employer wins, the community he serves wins, and his family wins.

Running into him was a shot in the arm and prompted me to follow up some of the other officers whose stories are in this book.

FRITZ: OFF IN A VERY NEW DIRECTION

Fritz was the young cop in Chapter 5 who left policing after he was nearly shot in the line of duty over the theft of merchandise worth $36. The shooting had created many cracks in Fritz's public persona as an easygoing tough guy. In our work together, he eventually related his current problems to growing up with an unpredictable, alcoholic father. After a while, he even came to think of his choice of profession as a mistake, part of his tough-guy image.

Today, Fritz is studying to be a set designer, giving full vent to an artistic side of himself that he had kept under wraps because it hadn't seemed macho enough. It's a low-paying job with a long apprenticeship at minimum wage, but it makes him very happy. It's been hard for him to go from a position of authority to being a student, but if someone offered him his law enforcement job back, he would say no without hesitation.

Fritz told me that he feels like an entirely different person. He describes himself as a "work in progress," by which he means he's dealing with a whole new set of emotions, as well as confronting feelings he has fended off all his life. "I lost so much of my real self as a cop. Cops always have a front up, and they can't drop it. Everyone pays—their families, their friends, and most of all they, themselves." He recalls how much he changed after the shooting, going from being low key to extremely aggressive in short order— a sure sign that he was under extreme stress. He laughs when he remembers that a lot of people said, "Cool, great, now he's getting it"—when, in fact, he was losing it big time.

On the downside, Fritz misses some of the drama he experienced as a cop. He finds drama now in his tumultuous love life, which seems as "wacky" to him as it is exciting. He catches himself still acting the role of rescuer with some of his lovers and sees how easily hooked he is by a female in distress—which is the role he played in his family, as well as in his work. He catches on earlier than he did before, but he isn't entirely beyond some of those old ingrained impulses.

Police work still intrudes upon his sleep. Whenever he is under a lot of stress, he has nightmares about being a cop. He dreams of the shooting or dreams he is back in a squad car, panicking because he can't remember what he is supposed to do.

He spends less time with his parents and has more emotional distance from them, which he thinks is good because they were too dependent on him. His dad is still unpredictable and given to rages; his mother is still victimized. But Fritz now takes all this much more in stride. He is less inclined to overreact to their emotional upheavals or to actively involve himself in their ongoing struggles.

I consider Fritz a success, although some might question his sanity for trading in a well-paid, secure position of authority for a low-paying career. I don't look at it that way. I applaud Fritz for making a number of positive but difficult moves.

- He was able to *let go* and move on when he determined that there was no way he could continue working as a cop without experiencing significant day-to-day distress.
- He used *introspection* and *self-reflection* to *confront* some

basic truths about his life, his upbringing, and his own character. That took guts.

- He wasn't afraid to take a *risk* and make a change—even though he didn't know what he wanted to do or if he could afford to do it.
- He *altered* his relationship to his parents, but he didn't abandon them.
- He developed a *process-oriented* view of life and doesn't expect to ever be finished evolving as a person.

STEVE: CALMING DOWN AND OPENING UP

Steve is the officer described in Chapter 2 who suffered from panic attacks and hypervigilance. His condition was so serious and disabling that he had to use several strategies to get back on track. He needed medication to overcome the disabling levels of anxiety he experienced during the initial crisis. He needed psychotherapy to confront layers of painfully unfinished business from his childhood. And he needed meditation and deep-breathing skills to stay calm and centered with and without medication.

His meditation practice has meant a great deal to him and his wife, Ginger. It fills a spiritual and social need and gives Steve something bigger than himself to use as a guide for living. He and Ginger have joined an organized group of meditators. They go to discussion groups and read Eastern philosophy. Their devotion to this practice has given them a new community outside of law enforcement, as well as something to share as a couple.

Ginger and Steve agree that his crisis was both the best and the worst thing that ever happened to them. Although it was incredibly frightening in the beginning, Steve is now more affectionate, involved with his children, light-hearted, and less controlling. He is more aware of his feelings and can contain his irritability and anxiety before he flies off the handle or before it snowballs into something unmanageable.

Steve has learned to replace negative thoughts with more positive or realistic ones. Until his panic attacks, he had no idea how conditioned he had become to negative thinking. Now he works hard not to overemphasize or dwell on gloomy, cynical, or grim thoughts. He practices positive self-talk and understands that his mind plays tricks on him, especially when he's under stress, and that with concentrated effort, he can quiet his mind and avoid getting panicky.

Meditating has brought Steve a new perspective. No longer is he the center of the universe. No longer does he indulge in what he calls "spectacular illusions": rescue fantasies in which he is the hero who saves the day and gets the medal. He doesn't need to be in the limelight or prove anything to anyone. It's okay for him simply to be good enough and to do what he's supposed to do. He understands he's not "God's gift to law enforcement."

For the first time in his 15-year career, Steve has applied for a promotion and a special assignment. He never dared do this before because he was secretly convinced he wouldn't get it, and he protected his ego by not trying. He had, as he says, "The easiest job in the organization—I was a critic." Now he's ready to take a risk despite occasional doubts that only "wusses" would look for staff work and real men stay on the street.

The biggest bonus is how much more involved Steve is with his family. He used to have a "love me or leave me" attitude. No matter how rude, preoccupied, or selfish he was, he expected Ginger and the kids to accept him. He left almost everything up to her, even though she worked full time. This made her feel like a single parent with two salaries. He always figured that the kids would get raised regardless of how much or how little he participated, and he literally didn't have time for anything else but his own insurmountable problems. Now he regrets having taken so much for granted. He understands how self-centered he was then and how important it is now that he attend to his children's moods and concerns—not the other way around.

Ginger also benefits from the changes Steve has made. She talks more openly about things that concern her in their relationship. She used to bottle things up a lot because Steve criticized her when she spoke out, telling her she was wrong for feeling what she felt. Now that he's more approachable, she's more open.

Things aren't perfect, of course. Ginger still thinks Steve is too caught up with himself, and she resents the time he spends with his hobbies. She has years of resentment to process and a lot of forgiving to do—some of it toward herself. She allowed Steve to make all her decisions and wishes now that she hadn't. She regrets not speaking up more when she was troubled. She wishes she had worked to be known and respected on her own merits and had not lived so much of her life through Steve. She wishes she had taken better care of herself instead of falling into the trap of taking care of everyone else first.

Ginger is tentative about the future, and her worst fears are that Steve will change back to the depressed and controlling person he once was. She doesn't worry about his job and never has. She thinks that most of Steve's problems were internal to Steve and that being a cop only fanned the already smoldering flames.

Steve's story, like the others, offers a hopeful message. There is help out there if you want it, both professional help and many self-help strategies. What it takes is determination to acknowledge and confront your problems rather than to deflect the blame elsewhere. It helps to have organizational support behind you—as Steve and Benny did—but people forge ahead without it when they have to, which is what Andy had to do.

ANDY: SADNESS AND SUCCESS

Andy was the jovial officer in Chapter 4 who experienced a significant personality change because of undiagnosed brain damage after an accidental head injury in a defensive tactics class. He retired on a medical disability after months of torment by some administrators who tried to charge him criminally and then fire him for threatening to shoot his commander. The mental health professionals who evaluated Andy concluded that his threatening behavior resulted from a delayed posttraumatic stress reaction and undiagnosed brain damage.

It's been a long haul for Andy, and he is only recently rebuilding his life. He and Dottie moved away, and no sooner had they done so than Andy's father fell ill with terminal cancer. Andy spent months commuting to his father's house until his father finally died. It was a depressing first year. He lost his father, his career, his friends, and his community—literally all that was familiar to him—over a very short period of time.

Andy now has a part-time job in the security department of a university, although he tried first to get work with local law enforcement agencies as a civilian property clerk or evidence technician. The hours are good, and the job provides the social contact he had lost, but he misses police work and the excitement of chasing bad guys. Sometimes he catches himself bragging about having been a cop.

What he misses most is the brotherhood. He tries to keep up with his old department, but this is difficult at a distance and he is no longer one of the gang.

Andy still has significant memory problems, and his forgetfulness continues to create friction between him and Dottie. Like Steve, Andy meditates and uses positive self-talk to keep from dwelling on things beyond his control, and he has been able to discontinue all his medication and psychiatric treatment. He still has emotional ups and downs—which are to be expected with the life stresses he has undergone and the brain damage he sustained.

Andy regrets what happened with his commander and wonders just "who that guy was" who made those angry threats. It sounds funny, but he can hardly believe it was he who did this. Occasionally, he dreams about the commander and about the shootings he was involved in. He thinks of his life as a movie and wishes he could reverse the reels.

Even with all his regrets, Andy has come to accept that it wouldn't be healthy for him to continue working as a cop. He has come to see policing as a young man's profession, not a lifelong career. If he had it to do over, he said he would have gotten the adrenalin rush out of his system and left after five years. When he watches cops working in his town, he sees the strain in their faces and remembers how much tension he had to bear between the far fewer exciting moments. He realizes that, beyond a temporary feeling of envy, he is really relieved to be doing something else.

Can a person be sad and successful at the same time? Of course. Andy lost a lot: abilities, potential, self-esteem, self-respect, friends, family, and security. It will take time for him to grieve his losses. His success lies in his resilience. He and his family have picked themselves up and moved on. Andy has not given into depression or bitterness. While he is mournful, he is not craving what he no longer has. He has been able to lay down new roots, make new connections, and envision a satisfying future for his family and himself.

LILLY: SOMETHING LOST, SOMETHING GAINED

Lilly left police work within months of shooting and killing the woman who was robbing her friend at gunpoint. At first she insisted on returning to work, believing if she couldn't do her job "the bad guys would have won." By "bad guys" she meant not just crooks but also all the skeptical cops who thought women weren't tough enough for this line of work.

Things were rough at home. The more Jack pushed to resume a normal life, the more Lilly felt abandoned and misunderstood. She experienced every request he made as a selfish demand and threatened to leave him.

Her sleep was disrupted with nightmares about the shooting. She was terrified of strangers and reluctant to venture out of the suburban community where she and Jack lived.

Two months after she returned to work she got into a "pissing contest" with a superior over something minor, tore off her badge, and left. She was angry and explosive with everyone. Her emotions were like an "avalanche," and she didn't have enough resilience to cope with even minor stress.

She felt devalued by her department—as though she were a used-up piece of equipment no one cared about. The chief had never acknowledged her bravery, and she yearned fruitlessly for his recognition. Instead of a commendation, she was written up for using sick leave to keep her appointments with me, and when she complained that this was unfair, she was written up for being angry.

Lilly was questioning everything and trusting no one. Should she stay a cop or quit? Should she leave Jack? She knew only one thing for certain—she could never again kill someone and survive. The shooting had left her feeling like "an egg without a shell."

She decided she couldn't work safely in the psychological state she was in and took a disability leave to concentrate on healing herself. She was consumed with guilt about the woman she had killed. She entertained ideas of trying to contact the family and apologize. She wanted them to know she was sorry and wished it had never happened. At night, her dreams were filled with images of mutilated corpses and bodies that wouldn't stay buried. She felt like a murderer.

Jack, meanwhile, was tiptoeing around at home, thinking that anything he did could make or break their relationship. He felt helpless and stupid in the face of Lilly's emotional turmoil—nothing he did was right.

Lilly remained in this painful position for over a year. She did everything she could to help herself: She took medication; had therapy once, sometimes twice a week; attended an anger management class; exercised; meditated; and learned to manage her panic attacks through desensitization, thought-stopping techniques, positive self-talk, relaxation exercises, and self-defense classes.

Gradually, things started to move. At the first anniversary of her shooting, she complained about not feeling stronger, but within months, she began to experience little successes—a trip into the city by herself or a night at home alone with no panic attacks. Her sense of humor returned. She had fewer nightmares. She began looking to the future instead of reliving the past. When she thought of the shooting, she could do so with detachment and compassion instead of guilt.

She started a group for other officers in similar situations. Starting this group was an incredibly healing step for her, as well as a service to others. It raised her self-esteem and showed her that she did have the ability to make a positive difference in people's lives, which was what had motivated her to become a cop in the first place. It gave her the opportunity to see how far she had progressed compared to others in the group—some of whom were raw with emotion in the immediate aftermath of their event; others who were still reeling from incidents that were years old.

Lilly never returned to work. She knew that as a cop she couldn't count on avoiding another shooting, and she was convinced she wouldn't psychologically survive a second. She was disillusioned by her agency's apparent lack of sensitivity to her situation and didn't have the heart to return to such an unsupportive work environment.

Few premature retirements go smoothly. Lilly had to fight for a settlement and a rehabilitation package. But she was able to focus her anger productively and find the energy to wade through the endless red tape and bureaucratic irritations. She retired, still waiting for a word from her chief.

After exploring several career directions, Lilly decided to open a home-based financial consulting business for women. She started by offering free classes at local recreation centers and adult night schools. Jack surprised her by printing up business cards, and he bought her a new computer and a fax machine. This was a wonderful gesture of support because he had as many misgivings about the financial insecurity of starting a consulting business as Lilly did about being financially dependent on Jack. They were both used to living well on two substantial and predictable paychecks a month, and now Lilly was bringing in half of what she had before and using that income for start-up money.

But Lilly was bursting with ideas and energy. She had a flair for marketing and teaching. It took only months before her business was booming, her client list growing, and she had more teaching requests than she could handle.

The transition from the public to the private sector has been challenging. Lilly has had to learn to live with the anxiety of being self-employed. She has had to develop the confidence to properly charge for her time, rather than to give it away for free, and to balance her commitment to providing affordable consultation for women with her need to earn a decent income.

As a businesswoman, Lilly feels as though she's discovering the real world for the first time; what she saw as a cop was only a small, grimy sliver. She feels liberated: No longer does she have to be suspicious of everyone and their motives; no longer does she have to be perfect.

Lilly and Jack still have their ups and downs. They had a fight on the second anniversary of Lilly's shooting, and in the midst of it, Jack let loose a torrent of feelings he had been keeping to himself. It is sadly ironic to see how the balance in their relationship is shifting. As Lilly's wounds are nearly healed, Jack is just starting to show his. As she grows stronger and happier, his unhappiness becomes more apparent. I could see from the beginning that they needed help as a couple, but couple counseling didn't appeal to either one of them at the time, although now it may. Jack made a common error—he assumed that

Lilly's problems were paramount and hoped that when she recovered everything would be back to normal. Nothing is ever "normal" after a fatal shooting—things may be better or worse, but they are hardly the same.

PHIL: A SEARCH FOR TRUTH

Phil, along with his partner, Bernie, was involved in the fatal shooting described in Chapters 5 and 6. Bernie was able to return to work with only minor problems, but Phil had a flashback on his first shift back and was placed on disability leave for several months and on light duty for several more. He spent nearly two years in counseling.

The shooting both frightened and infuriated Phil. He wanted his life back as it was before. Like Lilly, he was terrified of another shooting and the emotional aftermath. He overreacted to minor events and thought everyone was out to hurt him. He had near-panic reactions in shopping malls and parking lots. He avoided going out. His self-image as a fearless, always-in-control cop was shattered. When he returned to light duty, desk work left him exhausted. He was irate that this event had taken such a hold on him, angry with me for not having "cured" him during the debriefing, and fuming at himself for being "weak."

At home he was restless, irritable, and preoccupied. He had nightmares and couldn't sleep. He was claustrophobic and exercised fanatically to burn off tension. His fiancée, Trudi, tried hard to be supportive and understanding. But she had troubles of her own, and needed him for support as well. He recognized this need but he was unable to break out of his own misery long enough to help her. They grew distant, and their relationship buckled under the strain of their separate troubles. By mutual agreement, they sadly went their own ways.

Around the first anniversary of his shooting, Phil began reading philosophy—Plato, Aristotle, and Kierkegaard—as a way to soothe himself. He was on a search for the "ultimate truth" about what it meant to be a cop, what it meant to be a human being, and how best to reconcile the two. He was most confused about feeling remorse for a "scumbag" who had almost killed *him,* and he was "haunted" by the exchange of thoughts he had had with the suspect seconds before his death.

Phil had always thought of himself as an adrenalin-seeking, black-and-white-thinking cop with strong analytical skills. But all his intellectualizing couldn't make his feelings go away. He talked about how his soul hurt. The intensity of his feelings was so unlike anything he had previously experienced that he thought he was going crazy.

The logjam broke on the day he finally allowed himself to weep. All his life he had been trained to cover his feelings, and once that cover was gone, "little lightbulbs" went on everywhere. Incidents he had suppressed during 10 years of police work began to pop up and demand his attention. He started to value his emotions and his intuition, as well as his intellect. He began to reconcile the conflicts he had experienced by linking them together—it was possible to be tough *and* tender, courageous *and* cautious.

Phil's experience led him to start a peer-staffed, trauma response team in his department. He was determined to value in others what he had previously failed to value in himself—the emotional and spiritual side of his personality. He hoped to inspire others to take better care of themselves by revealing the details of his experience to spellbound coworkers in department-wide training on critical incident stress.

Today Phil is a more careful, cautious cop, who is unwilling to take unnecessary personal risks "for the thrill of it." He is no longer interested in impressing himself or someone else with his bravery. He paces himself better and is less driven. He is more a team player than a lone wolf. He again has a future in policing and the expectation that he will work a full 20 years before retiring.

Phil recently married. He says he is closer to his new wife than to any other woman he has known before. He thinks the shooting and the psychological work he did in its aftermath have made him a better mate—less guarded, more communicative, and more emotionally present to himself and the people around him. The shooting humbled him, forced him to get close to his own core; it showed him that his *soul* was not bulletproof, and it taught him that trusting others could soothe his most private pain.

272

DUKE: CLEAN AND SOBER

Duke was the alcoholic officer in Chapter 9 who went to pieces in a drunken rage. He voluntarily admitted himself to a psychiatric hospital and then to a 28-day residential treatment program. That was several years ago.

When you see Duke these days, he's cheerful, robust, and energetic. He's a peer support counselor, a member of the critical incident response team, an acting watch commander, the author of his agency's policy on alcohol and drug abuse, a new grandfather, and one of the remaining few residents of his treatment program who has *not* had a relapse.

He has written a journal about his recovery from alcoholism, which he generously shares. Like many recovering drinkers, he is dedicated to helping others. He is an especially credible role model for other cops, who know what he has been through and how well he's managing today.

Once Duke started dealing with his alcoholism, work stress, and depression, his son was able to have a life of his own. He no longer had to keep his father company or hang around the house to prevent him from killing himself. Paradoxically, they are emotionally closer since their tangled relationship has been straightened out and they each have separate lives.

Duke's drinking cost him two marriages and several relationships, including the one he was in when I met him. Even though he loves his children, while he was drinking he was beyond talking about the everyday domestic tasks necessary to raise a family. He was desensitized to all but the most violent, exciting events and didn't have any interest in ordinary conversations. He considers it a miracle that his children still love and respect him after what he put them through.

Duke is in a new relationship. He's confident that this time he understands what it takes to be a good partner, as well as a good dad. Like Phil and Steve, he's more humble and no longer expects the family to revolve around his needs. As inflated as it sounds, he was heartbroken at first to find out he was not the center of the universe. But now that he's been sober for some years, it feels like a relief.

Duke actively works on maintaining his relationships with friends and family: tending to them with time, talking things through, asking about feelings, and telling people how important they are to him and how much he appreciates and needs them. He knows from experience that he can lose his support system if he doesn't support it back.

SUMMING UP

What constitutes success or failure? The answer seems to depend on *whom* you ask and *when* you ask it. The officers and families described in this book have each defined their successes differently. Some of them made distinct choices, whereas others felt successful if they adjusted well to a situation over which they had little or no choice. For many, it was impossible to tell whether the decisions they made would turn out well until long after they had been implemented.

It is hard to define success and harder still to define a successful marriage or family. No outsider ever truly knows what goes on between two people, and it is a mistake to judge the quality of a relationship by its public face. An enduring marriage may not be happy or healthy. Some marriages work better for one partner than the other, depending on which mate you ask. We all know picture-book marriages that are privately abusive or families who bicker constantly but love each other ardently.

All relationships have their ups and downs. Young parents have to adjust to the numerous physical and emotional demands that children make. Middle-aged families have a different set of accommodations to make around physical and emotional losses. As the proverb says, "There is nothing so constant as change."

The families in this book have demonstrated how important it is to anticipate, accommodate, or perhaps even appreciate the inevitability of change. Their successes can be partially measured by their ability to attune themselves to change and to contain their anxiety over how much their lives have altered. Strength of commitment and the flexibility to adapt to hard times are paramount ingredients in an enduring, successful marriage.

The families in this book have a lot to teach us. Their stories contain some larger truths that can be generalized to police families everywhere.

- *There is more to life than the badge.* One of the greatest risks of police work is that cops become so inflated, narcissistic, and self-involved that they risk alienating their real families by overinvesting in the work family, which too frequently turns out to be fickle and unsupportive.
- One of the greatest risks to families is that they surrender their own identity in favor of the officer. In this book, the women especially have had a hard time focusing on themselves and later regretted losing that focus.
- *Families must come first.* The police department will be an insistent intruder into the family and must be dealt with effectively. Managing intrusions from the workplace is a critical element in building a family; this is especially the case for the many families in which both partners have full-time careers.
- The families in this book learned, some more readily than others, that scapegoating the job—or each other—doesn't help resolve conflicts. What did help was the ability to communicate with each other and work on solving problems rather than deflecting blame to the job or to each other. Families did best when they stayed focused on what they could control—time together as a couple, family activities, communication, finances, and long-range goals—and accepted what they couldn't control—occasional emergencies, traumatic incidents, shift work, politics, and bureaucracy.
- *What is risky is rewarding; what is rewarding is risky.* Accepting that police work is emotionally hazardous, the cops in this book almost always wound up learning how to better manage their psychological inheritance in order to better manage their psychological present. Many families stumbled and foundered because they had failed to come to grips with their families of origin and sometimes with their first marriages. They persisted in handling their adult relationships as though they were still seeing the world through the prescription glasses they had worn as children. Police work, in particular, seems to keep people in these old, rigid patterns, so both partners had to come to grips with the past in order to move on.

Cops in this book found an astonishingly wide range of tools to help themselves. They became master diagnosticians, learning to detect stress in themselves and their families. They broke free of old rescuer roles—which seemed to affect both mates and sometimes children—rejected rugged individualism, and accepted the need to ask for and receive help. Some learned to live with less than perfection in themselves and others. Most reset their expectations to a more reasonable, realistic level. Others started resisting peer pressure and started sharpening their ability to think for themselves. All seemed to find new, less self-destructive ways to burn off stress, anger, and adrenalin.

The people in this book have revealed a lot about the remarkable challenges facing ordinary cops and their families. They've shown how truly tough and resilient police families need to be to cope with an intensely challenging profession they have adopted only by proxy. They've disclosed what an achievement it is for cops to persist against heavy odds when they have been molded by a professional culture that values the short-range view over the long and action over introspection.

Their stories have exposed the continuing critical need for law enforcement agencies to invest in their employees' well-being and to value a durable family life as an integral part of what it means to be healthy. Almost all those cops who were treated patiently, respectfully, and compassionately were able to recover from massive psychological injuries and return to work. What cannot be calculated with any accuracy are the contributions these officers now make to their departments and their coworkers, both by their example and by their willingness to get involved with the teeming emotional life that percolates below the surface of almost any law enforcement agency.

I think the stories in this book also suggest that our law enforcement leaders need to rethink the traditional structure of police organizations and the traditional progression of a police career. Neither the promotional system as it exists nor the expectation of a viable 20-year career without promotion seems to be working for society or for individual officers.

EPILOGUE

The other day I was out with friends at a local urban festival. As we walked home in the early evening, large, boisterous crowds of teenagers lined both sides of the street and milled around a park. The atmosphere was spirited and tense at the same time. It felt as if the smallest upset—a look, a push, a flirtation—could spark a rampage.

All day, the cops had kept a low profile and joined the celebratory mood. They greeted people and asked if they were enjoying themselves. They smiled a lot, listened to the music, and sampled the food. It was a successful effort to avoid inflaming people with an overly militant police presence, but at the same time, it sent a clear message that the police were there and prepared to keep things safe and secure for everyone.

At dusk, the cops were still trying to keep a low profile, only now it was harder. They were outnumbered and surrounded on two sides by restless adolescents. They couldn't see into the crowd. There were few families or adults in sight.

Up and down the street, cops leaned casually on their patrol cars or talked quietly in small groups. Avoiding the crowd on the sidewalk, we stepped into the street and walked past a young officer who was standing in a relaxed posture, one foot on the bumper of his patrol car. As I got closer, I saw how edgy and apprehensive he really was, how his eyes constantly scanned the crowd. I felt like a spy. He was trying so hard to look cool and brave. No one was supposed to see his fear or concern: not the crowd, not his peers, not himself.

Later on, at home, we talked about how apprehensive *we* had felt in that nearly unruly crowd. Was it our imagination? Did we stand out as much as we thought we did? Were we in any danger? Talking defused the tension, and it was reassuring to know that none of us was alone in feeling and hiding a measure of strain.

I wondered about the young officer. I hoped that he, too, had the comfort and consolation of a loving family or close friends with whom to share the events of the day. I hoped he felt secure enough to talk candidly about the fear he had felt, as well as the fun he had had, and I hope he remembered to ask his family about their day as well.

RESOURCES

This section lists organizations, websites, books, and other sources of information to help police officers and their families. These listings have been updated and expanded for this revised edition and now include some resources outside the United States, particularly for Canada and the United Kingdom. In no case should any listing be taken as an endorsement.

The first part of this section is organized alphabetically under the following categories:

- General Psychological Support and Referral
- Trauma and Stress
- Grief Counseling, Victim Support, and Suicide Prevention
- Family and Couple Support
- Family Disaster Preparedness
- Alcoholism, Substance Abuse, and Gambling
- Domestic Abuse
- Other Support and Advocacy Groups (ethnic minorities, gays, lesbians, women, retirees, chaplains, self-help)

You'll find international resources within the categories under the heading "Outside the United States."

The second part contains recommended reading organized under these categories:

- Police Families and Family Life
- Alcoholism and Alcoholic Families
- Stress Management, Trauma, and Mental Health
- Special Families, Special Issues

- Spirituality
- Videos and DVDs

The Resources end with listings of publishers and other book sources.

GENERAL PSYCHOLOGICAL SUPPORT AND REFERRAL

American Psychological Association
750 First Street NE
Washington, DC 20002-4242
800-374-2721
www.helping.apa.org

The American Psychological Association sponsors a public website on which you will find guidance and information on many topics relating to psychological health and well-being for adults and children. There are referrals, resources, and a free brochure entitled *The Road to Resilience*. Also available is an online version of the Posttraumatic Growth Inventory, developed by psychologists Richard Tedeschi and Lawrence Calhoun. This 21-item inventory assesses posttraumatic growth and identifies areas you may want to explore further.

APA Disaster Response Network
202-336-5898
www.apa.org/practice/drnindex.html

A nationwide collaboration between volunteers from the American Psychological Association and the American Red Cross, the network provides free onsite mental health services for disaster victims and responding emergency personnel.

COP-2-COP
University Behavioral Healthcare/
University of Medicine and
Dentistry of New Jersey
151 Centennial Avenue
Piscataway, NJ 08854
866-COP2COP
http://ubhc.umdnj.edu/cop2cop/main.htm

This crisis intervention telephone help line for law enforcement officers and their families in New Jersey provides peer support, clinical assessment, referrals to mental health practitioners, and critical incident stress management. For assistance in starting a help line in your area, call the toll-free number.

Disabled Police Officers Counseling Center, Inc.
9662 Pennsylvania Avenue
Upper Marlboro, MD 20772
301-599-0190; 24-hour crisis line: 888-202-2772
www.dpocc.org

This nonprofit organization provides free counseling services (individual, family, group, and career) to any disabled, retired, or active police officer. Other services include a job bank, occupational testing and evaluation, career counseling, and information and referral.

Fire/Police Referral Network
660 Kenilworth Drive, #101
Towson, MD 21204
888-347-3765

This no-cost, nationwide referral program provides a referral to the closest licensed mental health provider with experience in counseling families, couples, and individuals affiliated with law enforcement and fire departments. Participating providers have been screened to ensure a documented professional commitment to individuals in these high-risk occupations.

Law Enforcement Wellness Association
P.O. Box 504
Elmira, OR 97437
541-935-2594
www.cophealth.com

The website for the Law Enforcement Wellness Association, dedicated to the physical and psychological health of those sworn to serve, has information on police suicide prevention, peer support training, and physical fitness.

National Mental Health Association
2000 North Beauregard Street, 6th floor
Alexandria, VA 22311
703-684-7722
www.nmha.org

This association maintains a 24-hour information and referral hotline.

National Mental Health Consumers' Self-Help Clearinghouse
1211 Chestnut Street, Suite 1207
Philadelphia, PA 19107
800-553-4539
www.mhselfhelp.org

As the word "clearinghouse" suggests, this is a resource for information and referral to mental health self-help groups and organizations throughout the United States.

New York Disaster Counseling Coalition
7 Dey Street, Suite 200
New York, NY 10107
212-582-8208
www.nydcc.org

This locally based coalition of 500 volunteer mental health professionals provides no-cost services (counseling, therapy, psychopharmacology, inpatient addiction treatment, couples workshops, and retirement services) to uniformed and civilian law enforcement personnel and their families in the New York City tri-state area. It plans to extend services to other locations.

Policepsych.com

This site is maintained by experienced police psychologist Dr. Susan Saxe-Clifford. Her "library of articles" covers a wide range of health-related topics.

POPPA (Police Officers Providing Peer Assistance)
26 Broadway, Suite 1640
New York, NY 10004-1898
212-298-9111; 24-hour helpline: 888-267-7267
www.poppainc.com

This independent, volunteer peer support network is committed to providing a confidential, safe, and supportive environment to New York City police officers and their families.

Outside the United States

Australian Counselling Association
www.theaca.net.au

This is an association of 2,500 counselors and psychotherapists. On its home page, click on "Find an ACA Counsellor" to search for a counselor in your area.

British Association for Counselling and Psychotherapy
www.bacp.co.uk

This association's mission is to provide an automatic reference point for anyone seeking information on counseling and psychotherapy in the United Kingdom. Go to its home page and click on "find a therapist" to locate help. It offers extensive links to help lines and health-related sites.

Canadian Psychological Association (CPA)
141 Laurier Avenue West, Suite 702
Ottawa, Ontario K1P 5J3, Canada
888-472-0657
cpa@resourcecpa.ca
www.cpa.ca

The CPA's website provides a gateway to psychological information and services throughout Canada. Click on the "Public" page to access helpful Q&As about finding a psychologist, what to expect, and general information about mental health.

TRAUMA AND STRESS

National Institute for Occupational Safety and Health (NIOSH)
1600 Clifton Road
Atlanta, GA 30333
800-34-NIOSH
www.cdc.gov/niosh/homepage.html
www.cdc.gov/niosh/unp-trinstrs.html

The NIOSH website features a page for emergency services responders to learn about traumatic stress. The page has a list of symptoms, links to other sites, and advice on coping at work and home.

Criticalconcepts.org
www.criticalconcepts.org

This site is maintained by police psychologist Dr. Daniel Clark, who has specialized in suicide and PTSD. It is informative and easy to navigate.

David Baldwin's Trauma Pages
www.trauma-pages.com

This award-winning website focusing on emotional trauma and PTSD has a huge reading list. Go to page 4 and click on "PTSD in police, fire, and EMS workers" for police family information.

Gift from Within
16 Cobb Hill
Camden, ME 04843
207-236-8858
www.giftfromwithin.org

This private, nonprofit organization is dedicated to those who suffer from PTSD, those at risk for PTSD, and those who care for traumatized people. It develops and distributes educational material, including video-tapes, articles, books, and other resources, through its website and maintains a roster of survivors who are willing to participate in an international network of peer support. Click on "articles" and then "police" for readings related to law enforcement.

International Critical Incident Stress Foundation (ICISF)
3290 Pine Orchard Lane, Suite 106
Ellicott City, MD 21042
410-750-9600; 24-hour hotline: 410-313-2473
www.icisf.org

The ICISF maintains a 24-hour emergency hotline that will put you in touch with a peer-staffed, public safety (police, fire, and EMT) critical incident team in your area.

National Center for PTSD (a division of the U.S. Department of Veterans Affairs)
802-296-6300
www.ncptsd.org

This website is an educational resource for PTSD and other enduring consequences of traumatic stress.

On-Site Academy
216-222 Mill Street
P.O. Box 1031
Gardner, MA 01440-6031
978-632-3518
onsiteacademy@resourceaol.com

A nonprofit, confidential five-day residential program for police officers and other emergency service workers who have been profoundly affected by traumatic stress, this program is facilitated by peers and police psychologists. The fee includes room and board and may be covered by your insurance. You can refer yourself.

West Coast Post Trauma Retreat (WCPR)
4460-16 Redwood Highway, #362
San Rafael, CA 94903
415-721-9789
www.WCPR2001.org

Confidential five-day residential programs for small groups of emergency responders are staffed by peers, mental health professionals with police experience, and chaplains. Residents receive individual and group counseling, educational information, and practical tools for dealing with stress, depression, anxiety, and/or PTSD. Fees include room and board and may be covered by insurance or worker's compensation. WCPR also offers a two-day program of support, education, and assistance to spouses and significant others.

Outside the United States

Australasian Society for Traumatic Stress Studies (ASTSS)
www.astss.org.au

ASTSS provides a forum for the understanding, treatment, and prevention of major stress and trauma in the Australasian region. It has an extensive list of links to organizations in the area and worldwide.

Canadian Traumatic Stress Network
www.ctsn-rcst.ca

The mission of this network is to advance traumatic stress services, education, training, public awareness, and professional development. Click on "useful web connections" for a broad list of Canadian resources.

UK Trauma Group
www.uktrauma.org.uk

This network of clinicians and other mental health professionals provides traumatic stress services. The UK Services page has annotated contact information for PTSD specialists throughout the United Kingdom. Also offered on the home page is a link to several helpful articles for families and caregivers of people suffering from trauma-related stress.

Victim Assistance Online
www.vaonline.org

A comprehensive on-line resource center for victim assistance, this site includes the Canadian Directory of Victim Services and a quick index to victim services worldwide.

GRIEF COUNSELING, VICTIM SUPPORT, AND SUICIDE PREVENTION

American Foundation for Suicide Prevention
120 Wall Street, 22nd Floor
New York, NY 10005
888-333-2377
www.afsp.org

The foundation provides support groups for people who have lost a friend or family member to suicide. Call for the location of local meetings.

Compassionate Friends
P.O. Box 3696
Oak Brook, IL 60522-3696
630-990-0010
www.compassionatefriends.org

An international support group for bereaved parents and siblings, 650 chapters in the United States provide support, referral, and information. Contact the national office for general information on bereavement, a complimentary newsletter, resource catalogue, and name and phone number of the closest chapter in your community.

Concerns of Police Survivors, Inc. (COPS)
P.O. Box 3199
Camdenton, MO 65020
573-346-4911
www.nationalcops.org

This highly regarded national organization is dedicated to reaching out to help America's police survivors. Contact the organization for the chapter nearest you. COPS provides peer support, legislative advocacy, information about benefits, a newsletter, scholarships, memorial week activities, and summer camp for children.

National Suicide Hotlines USA
800-SUICIDE (800-784-2433)
www.suicidehotlines.com

This toll-free hotline works 24/7. The website has online crisis support, information, and referral resources.

National Law Enforcement Memorial Foundation
202-737-3400
www.nleomf.com

The mission of this foundation is to increase public support for law enforcement by commemorating those who have died in the line of duty. Go here for information about National Police Week and the National Law Enforcement Museum.

National Organization for Victim Assistance (NOVA)
Courthouse Square
510 King Street, Suite 424
Alexandria, VA 22314
703-535-NOVA
www.try-nova.org

Providing support and legislative advocacy for crime victims, NOVA maintains a 24-hour referral service for crime victims other than domestic violence.

National POLICE Suicide Foundation, Inc.
8424 Park Road
Pasadena, MD 21122
410-437-3343; voice mail: 410-379-4814
www.psf.org

The mission of this foundation is to provide suicide awareness, prevention training, and support services to meet the psychological and spiritual needs of officers, their families, and survivors of suicide. The director, police chaplain Robert Douglas, is a former officer and the author of two books: *Hope Beyond the Badge: An Officer's Support Book* and *Death with No Valor.* Both books can be ordered on the website.

Officer Down Memorial Page
www.odmp.org

This nonprofit organization is dedicated to honoring America's fallen law enforcement officers by preserving their memories, photos, stories, and the stirring reflections of those who love them.

Parents of Murdered Children, Inc. (POMC)
100 East 8th Street, B-41
Cincinnati, OH 45202
513-721-5683; 888-818-POMC
www.pomc.com

POMC provides peer support for parents and family members by mail, telephone, one on one, in groups, or through literature. It sponsors a memorial wall and publishes a newsletter.

Suicide Prevention Help
http://members.tripod.com/~suicideprevention/index.html

This site provides advice on coping with suicidal thoughts or suicidal friends.

Tears of a Cop
www.tearsofacop.com

This website is devoted to promoting awareness of police suicide and PTSD.

Teresa Tate
2708 SW 48th Terrace
Cape Coral, FL 33914
askt8@resourceaol.com

Teresa Tate is the widow of a police officer who committed suicide in 1989. She has been trained in peer support and has started a network for survivors of law enforcement suicides. Email her if you need assistance or know a law enforcement suicide in your area.

Outside the United States

Care of Police Survivors (COPS)
www.ukcops.org

A peer-based, registered charity dedicated to helping families of officers who have died in the line of duty, COPS was founded in 2003 by a retired police officer and the widow of a slain officer.

Centre for Suicide Prevention
www.suicideinfo.ca

Based in Calgary, this nonprofit organization provides information, training, and research related to suicide prevention and crisis management. The "Are You in Crisis?" page has a wealth of information about how to cope with your own or a loved one's suicidal tendencies and how to quickly find help. It also provides a list of crisis centers in Canada, the United States, and internationally.

International Victim Services and Assistance
www.vaonline.org/vsu.html

This is a clearinghouse for worthwhile links to victim services and law enforcement services in Canada, Australia, the United Kingdom, Europe, and other points around the globe.

FAMILY AND COUPLE SUPPORT

American Association for Marriage and Family Therapy (AAMFT)
www.aamft.org

The AAMFT website has many useful articles about coping with family problems, as well as a directory for locating a marriage and family therapist near you.

Beside the Badge
P.O. Box 304
Tecumseh, MI 49286-0304

This organization provides information and fellowship for supporters of law enforcement officers.

Copnet and Officer.com
www.copnet.org and www.officer.com

Both these huge sites link to hundreds of other police-related sites, including those of interest to families.

Federal Law Enforcement Officer Wives
http://groups.yahoo.com/group/Fleowives

This is a confidential support and information discussion group for wives, family members, and other loved ones of current or retired federal law enforcement officers. It is particularly interested in supporting those who have contracted PTSD in the line of duty.

Fraternal Order of Police Auxiliary
National Headquarters
1410 Donelson Pike, A-17
Nashville, TN 37217
615-399-0900
www.grandlodgefop.org

The Fraternal Order of Police Auxiliary was founded in 1920. Its purpose is to support law enforcement. There are more than 4,000 family members nationwide and chapters in many states.

Gottman Institute
P.O. Box 15644
Seattle, WA 98115-0644
888-523-9042
www.gottman.com

The Gottman Institute is renowned for high-quality research-based marital therapy. Visit its website, where you can take a relationship quiz, read self-help tips, get information about couples weekend workshops, and find referrals to Gottman-trained therapists throughout the United States.

Handcuffed Hearts
www.handcuffed-hearts.com

This easy-to-navigate site has many features, including a directory of resources by state, links to other police family sites, and advice for starting a spousal group of your own.

Heavybadge.com
www.heavybadge.com

This website is maintained by police psychologists Gary Aumiller and Daniel Goldfarb. Click on the two family issue links for some good advice.

Hume Lake Christian Camps
800-965-HUME
www.humelake.org

This global ministry sponsors a yearly retreat for police couples at their lake resort in Southern California. Go to its website and click on "adult and family programs" for more information.

Loveacop.org
www.loveacop.org

This is a closed email discussion list for spouses, both women and men, of current, former, and retired law enforcement personnel. Bridging the gap between isolation and community, loveacop endeavors to provide a secure forum in which spouses can trade their secrets of coping, develop new friendships, and share in the give-and-take spirit of the list. It maintains an extensive list of links for spouses of law enforcement officers.

National Institute of Justice (NIJ)
www.ojp.usdoj.gov/nij

The NIJ has sponsored several programs for law enforcement family support. Go to the NIJ home page and type CLEFS (Corrections and Law Enforcement Family Support) into the search box to get to a list of programs and publications for law enforcement families.

National Network for Family Resiliency
www.agnr.umd.edu/nnfr/home.html

This network provides an extensive collection of information about family resiliency and resources aimed at building family strengths.

Police Families
www.policefamilies.com

This award-winning website was funded by a grant from the National Institute for Justice and awarded to Drs. Ellen Kirschman and Lorraine Greene. The site features referral information; guest psychologists; activities for children; an active message board; free, downloadable workshop outlines; and PowerPoint slides for family orientations and other educational activities.

Policewives
www.policewives.org

This site provides fun, support, resources, and friendship for families of law enforcement officers.

Policewives discussion group
http://groups.yahoo.com/group/policewives

This is a restricted list for police wives for sharing jokes, recipes, questions, and heartaches.

Police Wives Online
www.policewivesonline.com

This site was started in 2005 with the goal of becoming a national resource and support center for the wives, husbands, family, and significant others of law enforcement officers.

POWCA (Peace Officers' Wives Clubs of California)
www.powca.org

This statewide support group sponsors many activities, publishes a newsletter, and serves as a model for those who want to form their own support group.

Stepfamily Association of America
800-735-0329
www.saafamilies.org

This national self-help organization has local support groups, educational conferences, and a catalogue of books, tapes, and resources for stepfamilies.

Street Survival Seminars
Calibre Press
P.O. Box 115003
Carrollton, TX 75011
800-323-0037
www.calibrepress.com

This is a fast-paced, information-packed, two-day seminar for cops. Spouses and children over age 18 are welcome, although some material is graphic. Check online for locations and schedule.

Virtual Naval Hospital
www.vnh.org

This website is a gold mine of information. On the home page, click on "information for patients" and go to "Homecoming after Deployment: Dealing with Changes and Expectations." The information you'll find applies to everyone, not just military personnel.

Women Who Love Cops
http://groups.yahoo.com/group/WomenWhoLoveCops

This is a list for wives, mothers, sisters, and girlfriends of law enforcement officers.

Outside the United States

British Association of Counselling and Psychotherapy

See the listing above under "General Psychological Support and Referral, Outside the United States."

Canadian Police Wives

http://groups.msn.com/CanadianPoliceWives

This online support group for spouses of Canadian cops offers a great deal of information, along with discussion forums.

Couples Counselling Network

www.ukcouplescounselling.com

Members of this network have specialized training and experience in working with couples in all kinds of relationships: heterosexual, gay and lesbian, married, cohabiting, engaged, separated, or divorcing. You can find a counselor on the website or use the online counseling service.

Mensline Australia

General administration: +61 3 8371 2800
24-hour helpline: 1300 78 99 78
www.menslineaus.org.au

This organization supports men who are dealing with family and relationship difficulties, particularly a family breakdown or separation. Help is available by telephone 24/7.

Ontario Association for Marriage and Family Therapy

www.oamft.on.ca

This is the Canadian branch of the American Association for Marriage and Family Therapy, and it provides many helpful, archived articles dealing with marriage and family problems, as well as a referral directory for finding a therapist near you.

Police Wives

http://groups.msn.com/PoliceWives

This is an international online support group where wives and partners of law enforcement officers from around the world can meet.

Toronto Police Employee and Family Assistance Program
416-944-9123
www.employeefamilyassistance.torontopolice.on.ca

This is a confidential assessment and referral source for Toronto police officers and their families. Go to the website for interesting articles and a list of related sites and links.

FAMILY DISASTER PREPAREDNESS

Federal Emergency Management Agency
www.usfa.fema.gov

Click on "preparedness" for information about community and family preparedness, disaster planning, and keeping your family safe.

U.S. Department of Homeland Security
www.ready.gov

This simple-to-navigate website sponsored by the U.S. Department of Homeland Security provides instructions about preparing your family for emergencies, including terrorist attacks. Topics include how to communicate in a crisis and creating an emergency kit.

Outside the United States

Canadian Centre for Emergency Preparedness
www.ccep.ca

This website's "personal preparedness" page has a complete checklist for family disaster preparedness, along with links to other disaster preparedness and community response groups throughout Canada.

Preparing for Emergencies
www.pfe.gov.uk

This comprehensive site has information on how you can help yourself and others in emergencies. The site is easy to navigate.

ALCOHOLISM, SUBSTANCE ABUSE, AND GAMBLING

Al-Anon Family Group Headquarters
1600 Corporate Landing Parkway

Virginia Beach, VA 23454-5617
800-344-2666
www.al-anon.alateen.org

Al-Anon provides self-help services for families of alcoholics. If no groups exist in your area, the Lone Member Service can help you. Telephone or write for a meeting directory of Al-Anon and Alateen or a catalogue of the available literature.

Alcoholics Anonymous
P.O. Box 459, Grand Central Station
New York, NY 10163
212-870-3400
www.aa.org

Write or telephone for the time and place of a meeting near you.

Betty Ford Center
39000 Bob Hope Drive
Rancho Mirage, CA
800-434-7365
www.bettyfordcenter.org

The Betty Ford Center has extensive experience in providing residential treatment for police officers, although it does not have a specific law enforcement unit. They also offer programs in California and Texas for family members and children affected by addiction.

Gamblers Anonymous
P.O. Box 17173
Los Angeles, CA 90017
213-386-8789
www.gamblersanonymous.org

Write or telephone for the time and place of a meeting near you.

Marworth Alcohol and Chemical Dependency Treatment Center
Lily Lake Road
Waverly, PA 18471
800-442-7722
www.marworth.org/law_prog1.htm

Marworth's Uniformed Professionals' Program is designed to treat police officers and firefighters with substance abuse problems. Professional staff members are assisted by recovering law enforcement professionals.

Narcotics Anonymous Headquarters
P.O. Box 9999
Van Nuys, CA 91409
818-773-9999
info@resourcena.org
www.na.org

Call or email to find out about meetings in your area.

National Association for Children of Alcoholics
11426 Rockville Pike, Suite 100
Rockville, MD 20852
301-468-0985, 888-554-2627
www.nacoa.org

The mission of this group is to be an advocate for all children and families affected by alcoholism and/or drug dependence. Click on "affiliates" for activities in your area.

National Black Alcoholism and Addictions Council
5104 North Orange Blossom Trail, Suite 111
Orlando, FL 32810
877-NBAC-ORG; 407-532-2747
www.nbacinc.org

This is a nonprofit organization of black persons concerned about alcoholism and drug abuse.

National Clearinghouse for Alcohol and Drug Information
P.O. Box 2345
Rockville, MD 20847-2345
800-729-6686
www.health.org

This information-filled site is maintained by the U.S. Department of Health and Human Services' Substance Abuse and Mental Health Services Administration.

Peace Officers' Fellowship Starter Kit
Craig Perman Weisman, PhD
Employee Support Services Bureau
Los Angeles County Sheriff's Department
4700 Ramona Boulevard
Monterey Park, CA 91754

213-738-3500
cpwiesma@resourcelapd.org

If you or someone you know wants to start a peace officers' fellowship meeting (an AA group for cops only) in your area, contact Dr. Weisman. The starter kit contains tips, forms, and important information about organizing a fellowship group.

Outside the United States

Alcoholics Anonymous UK
National helpline: 0845-769-7555
www.alcoholics-anonymous.org.uk

Alcoholics Anonymous Australia
www.aa.org.au

Alcoholics Anonymous Canada
www.alcoholics-anonymous.org/en_find_meeting.cfm

These websites are portals for AA groups throughout the United Kingdom, Australia, and Canada, and each contains general information about the AA recovery program.

DOMESTIC ABUSE

Abuse of Power
www.abuseofpower.info

This website provides information for women who have been abused by intimate partners who are law enforcement officers or firefighters. The content includes tactics of abuse when the perpetrator is an officer, working with the justice system, personal accounts by survivors, and unique circumstances facing victims who work in law enforcement. The site is maintained by domestic violence advocate Diane Wetendorf.

Domestic Violence Self-Assessment Tool for Law Enforcement
www.quinnbenner.com

This 23-item checklist created by an experienced police lieutenant and counselor is designed to be used by police officers. Any of the items is an indicator of potential violence in an intimate relationship. The checklist is available from Vicki Quinn at the website above.

800-799-SAFE
www.ndvh.org

This is a confidential 24-hour domestic violence hotline. Visit the website for more information about the hotline and about domestic abuse.

Stopdv.com

Domestic violence expert and former police officer Anne O'Dell's website features an extensive list of resources and information.

Outside the United States

Australian Government Office for Women
800-808-863
24-hour help line: 800-200-526
http://ofw.facs.gov.au

If you need help, go to the website and, from the home page, click on "women's safety agenda" and then "domestic violence help" for the telephone numbers of confidential crisis help lines in your state or territory.

Battered Women's Support Services
604-687-1867 (accepts collect calls) or toll free: 877-392-7583
directservices@resourcebwssorg
www.bwss.org

Based in Vancouver, this long-standing organization provides counseling and community education. There are links to other support services for battered women in Canada.

Women's Aid Federation of England
General inquiries: 0117 944 44 11
24-hour help line: 0808 2000 247
www.womensaid.org.uk

This is an excellent website with lots of information in many languages. Click on "if you or a friend need help" for a list of local refuges, help lines, safety tips, help for your children, and much more.

OTHER SUPPORT AND ADVOCACY GROUPS

Gay Officers Action League (GOAL)
P.O. Box 1774
Old Chelsea Station

New York, NY 10113
212-NY1-GOAL
www.goalny.org

GOAL publishes a contact list of gay and lesbian police associations worldwide. Where no association exists, it will provide names of openly gay officers who want to start one and are willing to help other gay cops.

International Association of Women Police (IAWP)
c/o C. Mackie
5413 West Sunnyside Avenue
Chicago, IL 60630
www.iawp.org

IAWP publishes a quarterly magazine, *Women Police*. It has 14 regional branches and 30-plus affiliates in the United States, Canada, and the Philippines.

International Conference of Police Chaplains
P.O. Box 5590
Destin, FL 32540-5590
850-654-9736
www.icpc4cops.org

This pastoral ministry serves law enforcement officers and helps police agencies develop chaplaincy programs.

National Center for Women and Policing
433 South Beverly Drive
Beverly Hills, CA 90212
310-556-2526
www.womenandpolicing.org

This national organization, dedicated to increasing the number of women police officers and raising community awareness about the benefits women bring to policing, is also active in developing new ways of assisting domestic violence victims and stopping police family violence. It is open to sworn officers of all ranks, civilians in law enforcement, community leaders, public officials, and educators. It publishes a newsletter and sponsors conferences and training opportunities.

National Organization of Black Law Enforcement Executives (NOBLE)
4609 Pinecrest Office Park Drive, Suite F
Alexandria, VA 22312-1442
703-658-1529
www.noblenatl.org

This command-level organization, with memberships available to rank and file, publishes a quarterly magazine and holds an annual training conference, among other services.

Parents, Families, and Friends of Lesbian and Gays (PFLAG)
1726 M Street NW, Suite 400
Washington, DC 20036
202-467-8180
info@resourcepflag.org
www.pflag.org

PFLAG is a grassroots organization of more than 55,000 families, offering support, education, and advocacy. It publishes a quarterly newspaper and holds annual conferences.

SCORE: Counselors to America's Small Businesses
212-264-4507
www.score.org

This nonprofit organization is a resource partner with the Small Business Administration. It offers free in-person and online mentoring for anyone considering opening a business. It has 490 chapters nationwide. The New York City chapter has a model program to assist emergency responders who are facing planned or premature retirements and have unique challenges in reentering the civilian world.

Self-Help Clearinghouses
http://mentalhelp.net/selfhelp/
www.cmhc.com/selfhelp

These two websites catalogue self-help support groups and networks throughout the world.

Outside the United States

British Association for Women Police (BAWP)
07790 505204
www.bawp.org

The only national organization to draw members from all ranks and grades in the police service and associated organizations throughout England, Scotland, Northern Ireland, and Wales, BAWP aims to facilitate awareness of issues affecting women police officers, develop a network, share information, and contribute to the continuous professional development of all members. An extensive list of links is on the website.

European Network of Police Women
www.enp.nl

The mission of this network is to promote "quality through equality" by facilitating positive change in regard to gender, and diversity, as well as optimizing the position of women. It holds conferences and seminars.

Gay Police Association
24-hour hotline: 07092 700 000
www.gay.police.uk

This British-based organization works toward equal opportunities for gay officers, offers advice and support, and seeks to promote better relations between the police service and the gay community.

Police Federation of England and Wales
www.polfed.org

This is an information-packed website of an association headquartered in Surrey that represents the interests of 139,000 constables, sergeants, inspectors, and chiefs. Click on the "links" tab for links to regional police associations and special-interest groups for cops in the United Kingdom, including associations for policewomen and minorities.

RECOMMENDED READING

Police Families and Family Life

Aumiller, G. S. (1995). *Keeping it simple: Sorting out what really matters in your life*. Holbrook, MA: Adams.—A police psychologist offers a step-by-step plan for simplifying life. The book uses a lot of police humor and features the experiences of a troubled cop named "Mike" to illustrate the author's strategy for sorting out priorities and reducing stress.

Coughlin, A., Hern, S., & Ard, J. (1999). *You know you're a peace officer's wife when. . . .* (A project of the Peace Officer's Wives' Clubs Affiliated [POWCA] of California). Available from Davis Publishing Co., 1060

Calle Cordillera, San Clemente, CA 92673; lawtechpublishing.com; 800-498-0911. $7.50.—This little booklet, first published in 1978, has been updated. It was written by police wives for police wives and contains many helpful, wise suggestions.

Doherty, W. J. (2001). *Take back your marriage: Sticking together in a world that pulls us apart.* New York: Guilford Press.—The author helps couples pinpoint marital problems and take steps to stay close and connected. It is intended for happy newlyweds who want to stay that way and veteran couples on the brink of divorce.

Elgin, S. H. (1995). *You can't say that to me!: Stopping the pain of verbal abuse.* New York: Wiley.—Offers a step-by-step approach to dealing with verbal abuse and establishing a nonabusive language environment.

Finn, P., & Tomz, J. (1997). *Developing a law enforcement stress program for officers and their families* (NCJ 163175).—Available free from the National Institute of Justice, Washington, DC 20531.

Gilmartin, K. (2002). *Emotional survival for law enforcement: A guide for officers and their families.* Available from E-S Press, PMB 233, 2968 West Ina Road, Tucson, AZ 85741, or order online at www.emotionalsurvival. com.—Retired sheriff's deputy and psychologist Gilmartin has condensed his informative and successful seminars into book form. A must read for officers and families.

Gordon, T. (2000). *Parent effectiveness training.* New York: Three Rivers Press. This newly revised classic book on parent–child relationships is still useful today.

Gottman, J. M. (1994). *Why marriages succeed or fail: What you can learn from the breakthrough research to make your marriage last.* New York: Simon & Schuster.—Gottman describes the marriage styles and signs that indicate that a marriage is deteriorating and offers tips for improving the relationship.

Gottman, J. M. (1999). *The seven principles for making marriage work.* New York: Crown.—This book is packed with exercises and questionnaires for making your marriage work.

Grollman, E. A. (1991). *Talking about death: A dialogue between parent and child.* Boston: Beacon Press.—One part of the book is written for children. A second part is written for parents and addresses the kinds of questions kids are likely to ask about death. Contains an extensive list of referral sources and age-appropriate recommended readings and videos for children and adults who are coping with the death of a loved one by accident, illness, suicide, or homicide.

Lerner, H. G. (1985). *The dance of anger: A woman's guide to the changing patterns of intimate relationships.* New York: Harper & Row. Lerner, H. G. (1989). *The dance of intimacy: A woman's guide to courageous acts of change in key relationships.* New York: Harper & Row.—Both of these books are aimed at women, but I think they apply equally well to men. They are compassionate and filled with practical wisdom and understanding.

McKay, M., Davis, M., & Fanning, P. (2004). *How to communicate.* New York: Fine.—This book emphasizes the skills necessary for effective communication.

Norcross, J. C., Santrock, J. W., Campbell, L. F., Smith, T. P., Sommer, R., & Zuckerman, E. L. (2003). *Authoritative guide to self-help resources in mental health* (rev. ed.). New York: Guilford Press.—This book, written by mental health professionals, describes and evaluates self-help books and movies.

Perez, D. W. (1997). *The paradoxes of police work: Walking the thin blue line.* Incline Village, NV: Copperhouse.—Perez, a former police officer turned professor, has written a book to help new officers and their families anticipate some of the frustrations that will permeate an officer's life. It's a little academic, but he covers all the bases.

Quindlen, A. (1998). *Black and blue.* New York: Random House.—A realistic novel that was an Oprah Bookclub selection about an abused police wife.

Stone, V. (1999). *Cops don't cry: A book of help and hope for police families.* Available from Creative Bound, Inc., Box 424, Carp, Ontario, Canada KOA ILO.—Vali Stone is a writer married to a police constable in Canada. This book is a compilation of her personal observations and experiences, along with quotes from interviews she conducted during her research.

Sussman, J., & Glakas-Tenet, S. (2002). *Dare to repair: A do-it-herself guide to fixing (almost) anything in the home.* New York: HarperResource.— An illustrated guide written by two women whose husbands' law enforcement careers kept them away from home.

Tannen, D. (2001). *You just don't understand: Women and men in conversation.* New York: Quill.—A classic book about the differences in the way men and women communicate. This latest edition has a new afterword by the author.

Alcoholism and Alcoholic Families

Black, C. (1991). *It will never happen to me: Children of alcoholics as youngsters–adolescents–adults.* New York: Random House.—A powerful and insightful book for adult children of alcoholics.

Brown, S., & Lewis, V. S., with Liotta, A. (2000). *The family recovery guide: A map for healthy growth.* Oakland, CA: New Harbinger.—This book teaches family members how to sustain their relationships during a loved one's recovery from addiction.

Denning, P., Little, J., & Glickman, A. (2004). *Over the influence: The harm reduction guide for managing drugs and alcohol.* New York: Guilford Press.—This award-winning book is for those who want to cut down or gradually work toward sobriety.

Gorski, T. T. (1997). *Passages through recovery: An action plan for preventing relapse.* Center City, MN: Hazelden.—The author, an acknowledged expert in the field, explains how recovery works, describes six stages of recovery, and offers advice for working through the challenges of each.

Miller, W. R., & Muñoz, R. F. (2005). *Controlling your drinking: Tools to make moderation work for you.* New York: Guilford Press.—Shows drinkers how to become moderate drinkers by making small changes in their everyday behavior.

Stress Management, Trauma, and Mental Health

Armstrong, K., Best, S., & Domenici, P. (2006). *Courage after fire: Coping strategies for troops returning from Iraq and Afghanistan and their families.* Berkeley, CA: Ulysses Press.—If your officer has been deployed to war, this is the book for you. It is well researched, readable, and filled with practical suggestions.

Artwohl, A., & Christensen, L. W. (1997). *Deadly force encounters: What cops need to know to mentally and physically prepare for and survive a gunfight.* Boulder, CO: Paladin Press.—A police psychologist and a veteran cop teamed up to write a thoughtful, informative book about how cops can mentally and physically prepare for and survive a gunfight. Chapter 12 is devoted to families and trauma, but you'll learn a lot from the whole book.

Boorstein, S. (1995). *It's easier than you think: The Buddhist way to happiness.* San Francisco: Harper.—Short, down-to-earth book about Buddhist meditation applied to daily life.

Bourne, E. J. (2005). *The anxiety and phobia workbook* (4th ed.). Oakland, CA: New Harbinger.—Excellent source of practical information and help for those suffering from anxiety.

Davis, M., Eshelman, E. R., & McKay, M. (2000). *The relaxation and stress reduction workbook* (5th ed.). Oakland, CA: New Harbinger.—One of the most comprehensive stress management workbooks, it includes directions for mastering 14 self-care strategies such as time management, assertiveness, meditation, nutrition, and exercise.

Ellison, K. W. (2004). *Stress and the police officer.* Springfield, IL: Thomas.—A welcome second edition to this early classic. The author provides officers and administrators with individual and organizational techniques to identify and manage job-related stress.

Federal Emergency Management Agency. (1988). *Taking care of our own: Personal readiness guide for the responder's family.* Washington, DC: Author.—An excellent guide and workbook dealing with the psychological and practical challenges that occur before, during, and after long separations. It applies as much to law enforcement as it does to FEMA employees. Order this and many other family guides at usfa.fema.gov.

Goleman, D. (1998). *Working with emotional intelligence.* New York: Bantam Books.—This readable book demonstrates why emotional knowhow matters more than IQ at home and at work.

Greenberger, D., & Padesky, C. A. (1996). *Mind over mood: Change how you feel by changing the way you think.* New York: Guilford Press.—This write-in workbook is easy to read and understand. It will help you identify and then change the thoughts that contribute to your problems.

Hackett, D. P., & Violanti, J. M. (Eds.). (2003). *Police suicide: Tactics for prevention and intervention.* Springfield, IL: Thomas.—Strategies and tactics that may help to prevent police suicide.

Herman, J. L. (1997). *Trauma and recovery.* New York: Basic Books.—Beautifully written, deeply serious book about the aftermath of trauma.

Kabat-Zinn, J. (2005). *Wherever you go, there you are: Mindfulness meditation in everyday life.* New York: Hyperion.—A quick read about applying meditation to daily life.

Kates, A. R. (1999). *CopShock: Surviving posttraumatic stress disorder (PTSD).* Tucson, AZ: Holbrook Street Press.—The resource section in this book is exceptional. The author can be reached at P.O. Box 399, Cortaro, AZ 85652-0399; 520-616-7643.

Klinger, D. (2004). *Into the kill zone: A cop's eye view of deadly force.* San Francisco: Jossey-Bass.—The author is a sociologist and former police officer. His book is an oral history of 80 officers who, like himself, shot someone in the line of duty. It reads like a novel.

Matsakis, A. (1992). *I can't get over it: A handbook for trauma survivors.* Oakland, CA: New Harbinger.—Lots of practical ideas and advice for recovery. There is a special section for specific traumas like rape, domestic violence, natural catastrophes, car accidents, and combat, as well as an excellent resource section.

Matsakis, A. (2005). *In harm's way: Help for the wives of military men, police, EMTs and firefighters.* Oakland, CA: New Harbinger.—Practical advice for coping with the fear, anger, and loneliness related to your partner's high-risk profession.

Mills, J. W. (1982). *Coping with stress: A guide to living.* New York: Wiley.—This classic workbook is still one of my favorites. The author takes an in-depth approach to coping with stress. His methods are practical, realistic, and manageable yet broad in scope.

Regehr, C., & Bober, T. (2005). *In the line of fire: Trauma in the emergency services*. New York: Oxford University Press.—A readable, practical, well-researched guide that speaks to emergency responders and their families, as well as the mental health professionals and peer supporters who provide them with services.

Rosenbloom, D., & Williams, M. B. (1999). *Life after trauma: A workbook for healing*. New York: Guilford Press.—The authors guide readers toward reclaiming a basic sense of safety, self-worth, and control over their lives, as well as the capacity to trust and be close to others.

Violanti, J. M. (1992). *Police retirement: The impact of change*. Springfield, IL: Thomas.—A comprehensive book written by an experienced police psychologist and researcher, it is available only from the author at violanti@resourcebuffalo.edu.

Special Families, Special Issues

Bolton, K., Jr., & Feagin, J. R. (2004). *Black in blue: African-American police officers and racism*. New York: Routledge.—The authors interviewed 50 African American police officers to provide real-life examples of the difficulties and discrimination these officers face every day inside and outside the police station.

Buhrke, R. A. (1996). *A matter of justice: Lesbians and gay men in law enforcement*. New York: Routledge.—Stories of lesbian and gay criminal justice professionals, showing the similarities and diversity of their experiences.

Fletcher, C. (1997). *Breaking and entering: Women cops talk about life in the ultimate men's club*. New York: Pocket Books.—The author of *Pure Cop* and *What Cops Know* turns her sights to women in law enforcement.

Gold, M. E. (1999). *Top cops: Profiles of women in command*. Chicago: Brittany.—Intimate portraits of trailblazing women who achieved command positions in law enforcement.

Harrington, P. E., & Lonsway, K. A. (2007). *Investigating sexual harassment in law enforcement and non-traditional fields for women*. New York: Prentice Hall.—Guidance on how to investigate sexual harassment and take proactive measures like prevention and training.

Leinen, S. (1993). *Gay cops*. New Brunswick, NJ: Rutgers University Press.—The first book-length study of gay officers, by sociologist Leinen, a former NYPD lieutenant.

McNaught, B. (1993). *Gay issues in the workplace*. New York: St. Martin's.—A book to read and share with colleagues and employers.

Schulz, D. M. (2004). *Breaking the brass ceiling: Women police chiefs and their paths to the top*. Westport, CT: Praeger.—Mini-biographies of the trailblazing women who constitute a mere 1% of police chiefs nationwide.

Spirituality

Friedman, C. (2005). *Spiritual survival for law enforcement: Practical insights, practical tools.* Available from Compass Books, P.O. Box 3091, Linden NJ 07036.—Nondemoninational spiritual fortification for police officers and guidance for police chaplains.

God's word for peace officers. Available from Peace Officers Ministries at peaceofficersministries.org. or 877-487-1717.—This special edition of the Bible contains an introduction by Police Chaplain Stephen Lee, himself a former police officer.

Videos and DVDs

By their own hand: A film about police suicide. Produced by the New York City Police Foundation, Inc., 345 Park Avenue, New York, NY 10154-0037; 212-751-8170; www.nycpolicefoundation.org. $75.—This well-made training video is based on a study of police suicide and comes with an instructor's manual. It features candid interviews with officers who tried to kill themselves. The producers emphasize taking responsibility for one another and for getting help early.

Gay cops: Pride behind the badge. (2003). Available from the director/producer Charley Lang at www.Dakotafilmworks.com. $50.—An award-winning 30-minute documentary film about gay cops.

Homophobia in the workplace. Available from 800-876-7676.—An hour-long video featuring the humourous and gentle Brian McNaught, author of *Gay Issues in the Workplace* (New York: St. Martin's, 1993). He has unusual compassion for all points of view, even those opposing his, and he ties all his clearly stated issues to being able to work effectively and efficiently.

Stress management and the law enforcement family. (1994). Order online from the California Post Television Network (www.post.ca.gov/training/cptn/ordering.asp).—This video was originally produced as a telecourse. It includes candid interviews with police officers and their families, as well as several police psychologists. It comes with a workbook.

A tale of "O": On being different. Available from Goodmeasure, Inc., P.O. Box 381609, Boston, MA 02238; 508-883-2530; www.goodmeasure.com.—An animated video that looks at the experience of being one of the few, or an "O" among "X's." It explores the consequences of being different without finger pointing. Everyone can identify because everyone has been an "X" or an "O" at some time in life. You can see a video clip on the website.

BOOK SOURCES (PLACES TO BUY BOOKS BY MAIL)

Chevron Publishing
5018 Dorsey Hall Drive, #104
Ellicott City, MD 21042
410-740-006
www.chevronpublishing.com

Distributes and publishes books and videos about trauma and critical incident stress. Specializes in materials relevant to public safety.

Childswork/Childsplay
Center for Applied Psychology, Inc.
P.O. Box 615861586
King of Prussia, PA 19406
For catalogue: 800-962-1141
www.childswork.com

Childswork/Childsplay publishes and distributes books and games that address the mental health needs of children and their families through play.

Guilford Publications
72 Spring Street
New York, NY 10012
800-365-7006
www.guilford.com

A leading publisher of books for professionals and the general public about psychology, education, self-help, relationships, health, and parenting.

Hazelden Educational Materials
P.O. Box 11
Center City, MN 55012
800-257-7810; 651-213-4200
www.hazeldenbookplace.org

Check the website for a catalogue of books, pamphlets, and audio- and videocassettes about alcoholism, drug addiction, and other forms of substance abuse.

Impact Publishers
P.O. Box 6016
Atascadero, CA 93423-6016

805-466-5917
www.impactpublishers.com

Impact publishes and distributes self-help books.

MAC Publishing
321 High School Road NE
Bainbridge Island, WA 98110
800-698-0148
www.claudiablack.com

Recovery materials, books, and videos for adults and children written or developed by Dr. Claudia Black, an addictions specialist with a wide following.

Magination Press
magination@resourceapa.org
800-374-2721
www.maginationpress.com

Magination publishes books to help parents help their children. It also publishes *BRAKES: An Interactive Newsletter for Kids with Attention Deficit Disorder.*

New Harbinger Publications
5674 Shattuck Avenue
Oakland, CA 94609
800-748-6273
www.newharbinger.com

Publishes a wide variety of quality self-help books and tapes designed to offer step-by-step techniques for the reader.

Western Psychological Services Creative Therapy Store
12031 Wilshire Boulevard
Los Angeles, CA 90025
800-648-8857
www.creativetherapystore.com

Publishes and distributes board games, toys, books, and activities that assist children and families in coping with emotions, losses, stress, change, communication, self-esteem, and other challenging life events.

BIBLIOGRAPHY

INTRODUCTION

Bouza, A. V. (1990). *The police mystique: An insider's look at cops, crime, and the criminal justice system.* New York: Plenum Press.

Insel, S. (1994). Applying organization behavior principles to strengthen law enforcement families and reduce stress. In J. Reese & E. Scrivner (Eds.), *Law enforcement families: Issues and answers* (#1994-387-165/24333, pp. 287–295). Washington, DC: U.S. Department of Justice, Federal Bureau of Investigation, U.S. Government Printing Office.

CHAPTER ONE

Anderson, B. J. (1991, May 20). *On the front lines: Police stress and family well-being* (45-659-0-91-1, p. 99). Hearing before the Select Committee on Children, Youth, and Families, House of Representatives, 102nd Congress. Washington, DC: U.S. Government Printing Office.

Anson, R., & Bloom, M. (1988). Police stress in an occupational context. *Journal of Police Science and Administration, 16,* 4.

Bibbins, V. (1986). The quality of family and marital life of police personnel. In J. Reese & H. Goldstein (Eds.), *Psychological services for law enforcement* (85-600538, pp. 423–427). Washington, DC: U.S. Government Printing Office.

Bourne, E. J. (1990). *The anxiety and phobia workbook.* Oakland, CA: New Harbinger.

Coughlin, A., Hern, S., & Ard, J. (1978). *You know you're a peace officer's wife when. . . .* (A project of the Peace Officers' Wives' Clubs Affiliated, of California, POWCA). Montgomery, AL: Davis.

Davidson, M., & Veno, A. (1978a). Police stress: A multi-cultural, interdisciplinary review and perspective—Part I. *Abstracts on Police Science, 6*(4), 187–199.

Davidson, M., & Veno, A. (1978b). Police stress: A multi-cultural, interdisciplinary review and perspective—Part II. *Abstracts on Police Science, 6*(5), 257–268.

Flater, L. (1994). Officer/spouse workshops: A prevention and intervention technique. In J. Reese & E. Scrivner (Eds.), *Law enforcement families: Issues and answers* (#1994-387-165/24333, pp. 329–336). Washington, DC: U.S. Department of Justice, Federal Bureau of Investigation, U.S. Government Printing Office.

Greene, L. W., & Kirschman, E. F. On-line education, resources and support for law enforcement families. Final report. (Grant #98-FS-VX-0004, available at www.ncjrs.gov/pdffiles1/nij/grants/186749.pdf.)

Gordon, T. (1975). *Parent effectiveness training.* New York: Peter Wyden.

Janik, J. (1995, January). Who needs peer support? *Police Chief, LXII*(1), 38–41.

Kannady, G. (1993, August). Developing stress-resistant police families. *Police Chief, LX*(8), 92–95.

Maynard, P., & Maynard, N. E. (1982). Stress in police families: Some policy implications. *Journal of Police Science and Administration, 1*(3), 310.

McKay, M., Davis, M., & Fanning, P. (1983). *Messages: The communications skills book.* Oakland, CA: New Harbinger.

Niederhoffer, A., & Niederhoffer, E. (1978). *The police family: From station house to ranch house.* Lexington, MA: Lexington Books.

Scrivner, E. (1991, May 20). *On the front lines: Police stress and family well-being* (45-659-0-91-1, p. 99). Hearing before the Select Committee on Children, Youth, and Families, House of Representatives, 102nd Congress. Washington, DC: U.S. Government Printing Office.

Scrivner, E., & Reese, J. (1994). Family issues with no easy answers. In J. Reese & E. Scrivner (Eds.), *Law enforcement families: Issues and answers* (#1994-387-165/24333, pp. 3–7). Washington, DC: U.S. Department of Justice, Federal Bureau of Investigation, U.S. Government Printing Office.

Super, J. T. (1994). A stress prevention/intervention model for law enforcement officers and their spouses. In J. Reese & E. Scrivner (Eds.), *Law enforcement families: Issues and answers* (#1994-387-165/24333, pp. 375–384). Washington, DC: U.S. Department of Justice, Federal Bureau of Investigation, U.S. Government Printing Office.

Trompetter, P. (1986). The paradox of the squad room—solitary solidarity. In J. Reese & H. Goldstein (Eds.), *Psychological services for law enforcement* (85-600538, pp. 531–534). Washington, DC: U.S. Government Printing Office.

Whetsel, J. (1995, April). President's message: Honoring our fallen officers. *Police Chief, LX*(4), 6.

White, E., & Honig, A. (1995). Law enforcement families. In M. Kurke & E. Scrivner (Eds.), *Police psychology into the 21st century* (pp. 189–206). Hillsdale, NJ: Erlbaum.

CHAPTER TWO

Benner, A. (1993, March). Editorial. *San Francisco Police Department Peer Support Group Newsletter,* p. 2.

Bradstreet, R. (1994). Cultural hurdles to healthy police families. In J. Reese & E.

Scrivner (Eds.), *Law enforcement families: Issues and answers* (#1994-387-165/24333, pp. 19–26). Washington, DC: U.S. Department of Justice, Federal Bureau of Investigation, U.S. Government Printing Office.

Coughlin, A., Hern, S., & Ard, J. (1978). *You know you're a peace officer's wife when. . . .* (A project of the Peace Officers' Wives' Clubs Affiliated, of California; POWCA). Montgomery, AL: Davis.

Elgin, S. H. (1995). *You can't say that to me!: Stopping the pain of verbal abuse.* New York: Wiley.

Everstine, D. S., & Everstine, L. (1993). *The trauma response: Treatment for emotional injury.* New York: Norton.

Figley, C. B. (Ed.). (1995). *Compassion fatigue: Coping with secondary traumatic stress disorder in those who treat the traumatized.* New York: Brunner/Mazel.

Gilmartin, K. (1986). Hypervigilance: A learned perceptual set and its consequences on police stress. In J. Reese & H. Goldstein (Eds.), *Psychological services for law enforcement* (85-600538, pp. 443–448). Washington, DC: U.S. Government Printing Office.

Gilmartin, K. (1990). The brotherhood of biochemistry: Its implications for a police career. In H. E. Russell & A. Beigel (Eds.), *Understanding human behavior for effective police work* (3rd ed., pp. 397–418). New York: Basic Books.

Gray, J. (1992). *Men are from mars, women are from Venus.* New York: HarperCollins.

Hochschild, A. R. (1983). *The managed heart: Commercialization of human feeling.* Berkeley: University of California Press.

Honig, A., & White, E. (1994). Violence and the law enforcement family. In J. Reese & E. Scrivner (Eds.), *Law enforcement families: Issues and answers* (#1994-387-165/24333, pp. 101–107). Washington, DC: U.S. Department of Justice, Federal Bureau of Investigation, U.S. Government Printing Office.

Kirschman, E. (1983). Wounded heroes: A case study and systems analysis of job-related stress and emotional dysfunction in three police officers. *Dissertation Abstracts International* (University Microfilms, No. 83-19, 921).

Kirschman, E. (1994). Independence tolerance and dependence encouragement: What police agencies can learn from families. In J. Reese & E. Scrivner (Eds.), *Law enforcement families: Issues and answers* (#1994-387-165/24333, pp. 297–308). Washington, DC: U.S. Department of Justice, Federal Bureau of Investigation, U.S. Government Printing Office.

Lerner, H. G. (1985). *The dance of anger: A woman's guide to changing the patterns of intimate relationships.* New York: Harper & Row.

Lerner, H. G. (1989). *The dance of intimacy: A woman's guide to courageous acts of change in key relationships.* New York: Harper & Row.

Maslach, C., & Jackson, S. (1979, May). Burned out cops and their families. *Psychology Today, 12*(12), 58–62.

McKay, M., Davis, M., & Fanning, P. (1983). *Messages: The communication skills book.* Oakland, CA: New Harbinger.

Mills, J. W. (1982). *Coping with stress.* New York: Wiley.

Niederhoffer, A. (1976). *The ambivalent force: Perspectives on the police* (2nd ed.). New York: Holt, Rinehart, and Winston.

Philpot, C., & Borum, R. (1993). Therapy with law enforcement couples: Clinical management of the high risk lifestyle. *American Journal of Family Therapy, 21*(2), 122–135.

Satir, V. (1983). *Conjoint family therapy* (3rd ed., rev.). Palo Alto, CA: Science and Behavior Books.

Scrivner, E. (1991, May 20). *On the front lines: Police stress and family well-being* (45-659-0-91-1, p. 99). Hearing before the Select Committee on Children, Youth and Families, House of Representatives, 102nd Congress. Washington, DC: U.S. Government Printing Office.

Shapiro, E. R., & Carr, A. W. (1991). *Lost in familiar places: Creating new connections between the individual and society.* New Haven, CT: Yale University Press.

Territo, L., & Vetter, H. (1981). Stress and police personnel. *Journal of Police Science and Administration, 9*(2), 195–208.

CHAPTER THREE

Beck, A. T. (1988). *Love is never enough.* New York: Harper & Row.

Blau, T. H. (1994). *Psychological services for law enforcement.* New York: Wiley.

Bonifacio, P. (1991). *The psychological effects of police work: A psychodynamic approach.* New York: Plenum Press.

Bouza, A., (1990). *The police mystique: An insider's look at cops, crime, and the criminal justice system.* New York: Plenum Press.

Coughlin, A., Hern, S., & Ard, J. (1978). *You know you're a peace officer's wife when. . . .* (A project of the Peace Officers' Wives' Clubs Affiliated, of California, POWCA). Montgomery, AL: Davis.

Davidson, M., & Veno, A. (1978a). Police stress: A multi-cultural, interdisciplinary review and perspective—Part I. *Abstracts on Police Science, 6*(4), 187–199.

Davidson, M., & Veno, A. (1978b). Police stress: A multi-cultural, interdisciplinary review and perspective—Part II. *Abstracts on Police Science, 6*(5), 257–268.

Depue, R. (1981, August). High risk lifestyle: The police family. *FBI Law Enforcement Bulletin, 50*(8), 7–13.

Edelwich, J., & Brodsky, A. (1981). Expectations vs. limitations linking training interventions to needs on and off the job. In W. S. Paine (Ed.), *Proceedings of the First National Conference on Burnout* (pp. 197–226). Philadelphia: Mercy Catholic Medical Center.

Foreman, W. (1991). Police stress response to a civilian aircraft disaster. In J. Reese, J. Horn, & C. Dunning (Eds.), *Critical incidents in policing* (pp. 85–94). Washington, DC: U.S. Government Printing Office.

Gershon, R., Lin, S., & Li, X. (2002). Work stress in aging police officers. *Journal of Occupational and Environmental Medicine, 44*, 160–167.

Gilmartin, K. (1986). Hypervigilance: A learned perceptual set and its consequences on police stress. In J. Reese & H. Goldstein (Eds.), *Psychological services for law enforcement* (pp. 443–448). Washington, DC: U.S. Government Printing Office.

Bibliography

Grossman, I. (1994). Peter's other principle. In J. Reese & E. Scrivner (Eds.), *Law enforcement families: Issues and answers* (#1994-387-165/24333, pp. 281–286). Washington, DC: U.S. Department of Justice, Federal Bureau of Investigation, U.S. Government Printing Office.

Institute for Local Self-Government. (1977a). *Alternatives to traditional public safety delivery systems.* Berkeley, CA: Author.

Institute for Local Self-Government. (1977b). *Equity eroded: The disintegration of worker's compensation policies.* Berkeley, CA: Author.

Inwald, R. (1994). Three studies of police spouse/mate relationships using the Hilson Spouse/Mate Inventory. In J. Reese & E. Scrivner (Eds.), *Law enforcement families: Issues and answers* (#1994-387-165/24333, pp. 35–40). Washington, DC: U.S. Department of Justice, Federal Bureau of Investigation, U.S. Government Printing Office.

Jackson, S. (1983). Managing stress and burnout in law enforcement agencies. *R.C.M.P. Gazette, 45*(10), 2025.

Kaslof, L. (n.d.). *Advances, 6*(1), 20–21.

Lerner, H. G. (1989). *The dance of intimacy: A woman's guide to courageous acts of change in key relationships.* New York: Harper & Row.

Maslach, C. (1976, September). Burned out. *Human Behavior, 5*(9), 16–22.

Maslach, C. (1982). *Burnout: The cost of caring.* New York: Prentice Hall.

Maslach, C., & Jackson, S. (1979, May). Burned out cops and their families. *Psychology Today, 12*(12), 58–62.

Mitchell, J. T., & Everly, G. S., Jr. (1994). *Human elements training for emergency services, public safety, and disaster personnel.* Ellicott City, MD: Chevron.

Pines, A., & Silbert, M. (1980). *Burnout of officers. Study of the San Francisco Police Department.* Unpublished report.

Reaves, B. (1996). *Local police departments, 1993* (NCJ-160802). Annapolis Junction, MD: Bureau of Justice Statistics, U.S. Department of Justice Statistics Clearinghouse.

Reiser, M. (1982). *Police psychology: Collected papers.* Los Angeles: LEHI.

Saxe, S., & Fabricatore, J. (1982, August). Using psychological consultants in screening police applicants. *FBI Law Enforcement Bulletin,* pp. 8–11.

Scrivner, E. (1991, May 20). *On the front lines: Police stress and family well-being* (45-659-0-91-1, p. 99). Hearing before the Select Committee on Children, Youth, and Families, House of Representatives, 102nd Congress. Washington, DC: U.S. Government Printing Office.

Sheehy, G. (1976). *Passages: Predictable crises of adult life.* New York: Dutton.

Swanson, K. (1979). *Success without promotion.* Unpublished manuscript. (Available from the author, P.O. Box 8039, Walnut Creek, CA 94596)

Violanti, J. (1983). Stress patterns in police work: A longitudinal study. *Journal of Police Science and Administration, 11*(2), 211–216.

Violanti, J. M. (1992). *Police retirement: The impact of change.* Springfield, IL: Thomas.

Wallerstein, J. S., & Blakeslee, S. (1995). *The good marriage: How and why love lasts.* Boston: Houghton Mifflin.

CHAPTER FOUR

Bourne, E. J. (1990). *The anxiety and phobia workbook*. Oakland, CA: New Harbinger.

Bouza, A. V. (1990). *The police mystique: An insider's look at cops, crime, and the criminal justice system*. New York: Plenum Press.

Danto, B. L. (1979). Police stress—its causes and types. *Police Product News, 3*(10), 56–60.

Elgin, S. H. (1995). *You can't say that to me: Stopping the pain of verbal abuse—an 8-step program*. New York: Wiley.

Gilmartin, K. (1986). Hypervigilance: A learned perceptual set and its consequences on police stress. In J. Reese & H. Goldstein (Eds.), *Psychological services for law enforcement* (pp. 443–448). Washington, DC: U.S. Government Printing Office.

Jackson, S. E. (1983). Managing stress and burnout in law enforcement agencies. *R.C.M.P. Gazette, 45*(10), 2025.

Kirschman, E. (1983). Wounded heroes: A case study and systems analysis of job-related stress and emotional dysfunction in three police officers. *Dissertation Abstracts International* (University Microfilms, No. 83-19, 921).

Kirschman, E. (1987). Organization development: Buddha in search of the barrel. In H. W. More & P. C. Unsinger (Eds.), *Police managerial use of psychology and psychologists*. Springfield, IL: Thomas.

Kirschman, E. (1995). Law enforcement consultation: A view from the field. In M. I. Kurke & E. M. Scrivner (Eds.), *Police psychology into the 21st century* (pp. 375–390). Hillsdale, NJ: Erlbaum.

Kirschman, E. (1996). The psychologist as all-purpose housemother: Recommended attributes for the successful organization consultant. In J. Reese & R. Solomon (Eds.), *Organizational issues in law enforcement* (#1996-405-035/54337, pp. 155–164). Washington, DC: U.S. Government Printing Office.

Kirschman, E., Scrivner, E., Ellison, K., & Marcy, C. (1992). Work and well-being: Lessons from law enforcement. In J. C. Quick, L. R. Murphy, & J. J. Hurrell, Jr. (Eds.), *Stress and well-being at work: Assessments and interventions for occupational mental health* (pp. 178–192). Washington, DC: American Psychological Association.

Kirschman, E., & Walima, S. (1988, October). Health resource coordinators: Organization consultation services. *Police Chief, LV*(10), 78–82.

Kramer, M. (1974). *Reality shock*. St. Louis, MO: Mosby.

Kroes, W., & Gould, S. (1979). Job stress in policemen; an empirical study. *Police Stress, 1*(2), 10, 44–46.

Kroes, W., & Hurrell, J. (1974). *Job stress and the police officer*. Washington, DC: U.S. Government Printing Office.

Lerner, H. G. (1985). *The dance of anger: A woman's guide to changing the patterns of intimate relationships*. New York: Harper & Row.

Maynard, P., & Maynard, N. (1982). Stress in police families: Some policy implications. *Journal of Police Science and Administration, 10*(3), 302–314.

McKay, M., Davis, M., & Fanning, P. (1983). *Messages: The communication skills book*. Oakland, CA: New Harbinger.

White, E., & Honig, A. (1995). Law enforcement families. In M. I. Kurke & E. M. Scrivner (Eds.), *Police psychology into the 21st century* (pp. 189–206). Hillsdale, NJ: Erlbaum.

CHAPTER FIVE

American Psychiatric Association. (1994). *Diagnostic and statistical manual of mental disorders* (4th ed.). Washington, DC: Author.

Baum, D. (2006, January 9). Deluged: The New Orleans police and Katrina. *The New Yorker*.

Calhoun, L., & Tedeschi, R. (2000). Early posttraumatic interventions: Facilitating possibilities for growth. In J. M. Violanti, D. Paton, & C. Dunning (Eds.), *Posttraumatic stress intervention: Challenges, issues, and perspectives* (pp. 135–152). Springfield, IL: Thomas.

Everstine, D. S., & Everstine, L. (1993). *The trauma response: Treatment for emotional injury*. New York: Norton.

Figley, C. R. (1995). *Compassion fatigue: Coping with secondary traumatic stress disorder in those who treat the traumatized*. New York: Brunner/Mazel.

IACP News. (1997). *Police Chief, LXIV*(2), 61.

King, L. (2000, Spring). *The power of belief: Thoughts that harm, thoughts that heal*. Lecture presented at the Institute for CorTexT Research and Development, Oakland, CA.

Kirschman, E. (1994). Independence tolerance and dependence encouragement: What police agencies can learn from families. In J. Reese & E. Scrivner (Eds.), *Law enforcement families: Issues and answers* (#1994-387-165/24333, pp. 297–308). Washington, DC: U.S. Department of Justice, Federal Bureau of Investigation, U.S. Government Printing Office.

Kirschman, E. (2004). *I love a fire fighter: What the family needs to know*. New York: Guilford Press.

Maguire, K., & Pastore, A. (Eds.). (1995). *Sourcebook of criminal justice statistics—1994* (NCJ-154591). Washington, DC: U.S. Department of Justice, Bureau of Justice Statistics, U.S. Government Printing Office.

Marmar, C., Best, S., Metzler, T., Chemtob, C., Gloria, R., Killeen, A., et al. (2003, July 11). *Impact of the World Trade Center attacks on New York City police officers*. Invited grand rounds presentation, Department of Psychiatry, Columbia University, New York.

Matsakis, A. (1992). *I can't get over it: A handbook for trauma survivors*. Oakland, CA: New Harbinger.

Mitchell, J. T., & Everly, G. S., Jr. (1993). *Critical incident stress debriefing: An operations manual for the prevention of traumatic stress among emergency service and disaster workers*. Ellicott City, MD: Chevron.

Quereshi, K., Gershon, R. R., Sherman, M. F., Straub, T., Gebbie, E., McCollum, M., et al. (2005). Health care workers' ability and willingness to report to duty during catastrophic disasters. *Journal of Urban Health: Bulletin of the New York Academy of Medicine, 82*(3), 378–388.

Regehr, C., & Bober, T. (2005). *In the line of fire: Trauma in the emergency services.* New York: Oxford University Press.

Solomon, R., & Horn, J. (1986). Post shooting traumatic reactions: A pilot study. In J. Reese & H. Goldstein (Eds.), *Psychological services for law enforcement* (85-600538, pp. 383–394). Washington, DC: U.S. Government Printing Office.

Terkel, S. (1972). *Working.* New York: Avon Books.

Trompetter, P. (1994). Assessing the psychological well-being of returning officers following a critical incident. *Journal of California Law Enforcement, 27*(3), 82–86.

Uniform Crime Report. (2004). Available at www.fbi.gov/ucr/cius_04

Ussery, W. J., & Waters. J. A. (2006, January). COP-2-COP hotlines: Programs to address the needs of first responders and their families. *Brief Treatment and Crisis Intervention, 6*(1), 66–78.

van der Kolk, B. A. (Ed.). (1987). *Psychological trauma.* Washington, DC: American Psychiatric Press.

van der Kolk, B. A. (1991). The psychological processing of traumatic events: The personal experience of posttraumatic stress disorder. In J. Reese, J. Horn, & C. Dunning (Eds.), *Critical incidents in policing* (pp. 359–364). Washington, DC: U.S. Government Printing Office.

Violanti, J. (1991). Posttrauma vulnerability: A proposed model. In J. Reese, J. Horn, & C. Dunning (Eds.), *Critical incidents in policing* (pp. 365–372). Washington, DC: U.S. Government Printing Office.

Violanti, J. M., Paton, D., & Dunning, C. (Eds.). (2000). *Posttraumatic stress intervention: Challenges, issues and perspectives.* Springfield, IL: Thomas.

Wilzcak, C. (2006). Gender differences in NYCPD work stress and trauma: September 11th 2001 and its aftermath. In J. M. Violanti & D. Paton (Eds.), *Who gets PTSD?: Issues of posttraumatic stress vulnerability* (pp. 50–69). Springfield, IL: Thomas.

CHAPTER SIX

Baruth, C. (1986). Pre-critical incident involvement by psychologist. In J. Reese & H. Goldstein (Eds.), *Psychological services for law enforcement* (85-600538, pp. 305–309). Washington, DC: U.S. Government Printing Office.

Figley, C. R. (Ed.). (1985). *Trauma and its wake: The study and treatment of PTSD.* New York: Brunner/Mazel.

Figley, C. R. (Ed.). (1986). *Trauma and its wake: Volume II. Traumatic stress, theory, research, and intervention.* New York: Brunner/Mazel.

Greller, M., Parsons, C., & Michael, D. (1992). Additive effects and beyond: Occupational stressors and social buffers in a police organization. In J. C. Quick, L. R. Murphy, & J. J. Hurrell, Jr. (Eds.), *Stress and well-being at work: Assessments and interventions for occupational mental health* (pp. 33–47). Washington, DC: American Psychological Association.

Bibliography

Herman, J. L. (1992). *Trauma and recovery: The aftermath of violence from domestic abuse to political terror.* New York: Basic Books.

Horn, J. (1991). Critical incidents for law enforcement officers. In J. Reese, J. Horn, & C. Dunning (Eds.), *Critical incidents in policing* (pp. 143-148). Washington, DC: U.S. Government Printing Office.

Johnston, C. J. (Speaker). (1996, May 3-5). *Welcoming address.* New York State Police Academy Symposium on Domestic Violence in Law Enforcement Families, Albany, NY.

Kabat-Zinn, J. (1990). *Full catastrophe living: Using the wisdom of your body and mind to face stress, pain, and illness.* New York: Delta Publishing.

Kirschman, E., Scrivner, E., Ellison, K., & Marcy, C. (1992). Work and well-being: Lessons from law enforcement. In J. Quick, L. Murphy, & J. Hurrell (Eds.), *Stress and well-being at work: Assessments and interventions for occupational mental health* (pp. 178–192). Washington, DC: American Psychological Association.

Klinger, D. (2004). *Police response to officer involved shootings: A report (97-IJ-CX-0029) funded by the Office of Justice Programs, National Institute of Justice, Washington, DC.* Available online at www.killzonevoices.com/default.php?pageID=reports&navID=3

Niederhoffer, A., & Niederhoffer, E. (1978). *The police family: From station house to ranch house.* Lexington, MA: Lexington Books.

Reese, J. (1987). *A history of police psychological services.* Washington, DC: U.S. Government Printing Office.

Regehr, C., & Bober, T. (2005). *In the line of fire: Trauma in the emergency services.* New York: Oxford University Press.

Shapiro, E., & Carr, W. (1991). *Lost in familiar places: Creating new connections between the individual and society.* New Haven, CT: Yale University Press.

Shapiro, F. (1995). *Eye movement desensitization and reprocessing.* New York: Guilford Press.

Solomon, R., & Horn, J. (1986). Post shooting traumatic reactions: A pilot study. In J. Reese & H. Goldstein (Eds.), *Psychological services for law enforcement* (85-600538, pp. 383–394). Washington, DC: U.S. Government Printing Office.

Trompetter, P. (1986). The paradox of the squad room—solitary solidarity. In J. Reese & H. Goldstein (Eds.), *Psychological services for law enforcement* (85-600538, pp. 531–534). Washington, DC: U.S. Government Printing Office.

van der Kolk, B. A. (Ed.). (1987). *Psychological trauma.* Washington, DC: American Psychiatric Press.

Violanti, J. (1991). Posttrauma vulnerability: A proposed model. In J. Reese, J. M. Horn, & C. Dunning (Eds.), *Critical incidents in policing* (pp. 365–372). Washington, DC: U.S. Government Printing Office.

Wambaugh, J. (1973). *The onion field.* New York: Delacorte.

Wessley, S. (2005, August 11). Victimhood and resilience. *New England Journal of Medicine.*

CHAPTER SEVEN

Centre for Living with Dying. (1987). *Living with trauma.* (Available from the author/publisher at 554 Mansion Park Drive, Santa Clara, CA 95054, 408-980-9801)

Danieli, Y. (1985). The treatment and prevention of long-term effects and intergenerational transmission of victimization: A lesson from holocaust survivors and their children. In C. Figley (Ed.), *Trauma and its wake: The study and treatment of PTSD* (pp. 295–313). New York: Brunner/Mazel.

Figley, C. R. (Ed.). (1985). *Trauma and its wake: The study and treatment of PTSD.* New York: Brunner/Mazel.

Figley, C. R. (1995). *Compassion fatigue: Coping with secondary traumatic stress disorder in those who treat the traumatized.* New York: Brunner/Mazel.

Gross-Farina, S. (1993, March). Fit for duty?: Cops, choir practice and another chance for healing. *University of Miami Law Review, 47*(4), 1110–1111.

Herman, J. L. (1992). *Trauma and recovery: The aftermath of violence from domestic abuse to political terror.* New York: Basic Books.

Kirschman, E. (1983). Wounded heroes: A case study and systems analysis of job-related stress and emotional dysfunction in three police officers. *Dissertation Abstracts International* (University Microfilms, No. 83-19, 921).

Lerner, H. G. (1985). *The dance of anger: A woman's guide to changing the patterns of intimate relationships.* New York: Harper & Row.

McKay, M., Davis, M., & Fanning, P. (1983). *Messages: The communications skills book.* Oakland, CA: New Harbinger.

Meichenbaum, D. (1994). *A clinical handbook/practical therapist manual for assessing and treating adults with PTSD.* Waterloo, ON: Institute Press.

Ryan, A., & Brewster, M. E. (1994). Posttraumatic stress disorder and related symptoms in traumatized police officers and their spouses/mates. In J. Reese & E. Scrivner (Eds.), *Law enforcement families: Issues and answers* (#1994-387-165/24333, pp. 217–225). Washington, DC: U.S. Department of Justice, Federal Bureau of Investigation, U.S. Government Printing Office.

Shapiro, E. R., & Carr, A. W. (1991). *Lost in familiar places: Creating new connections between the individual and society.* New Haven, CT: Yale University Press.

Tannen, D. (1990). *You just don't understand me.* New York: Morrow.

U.S. Department of Health and Human Services. (1987). *Prevention and control of stress among emergency workers* (Publication No. ADM 87-1497). Washington, DC: U.S. Department of Health and Human Services, Alcohol, Drug Abuse and Mental Health Administration.

CHAPTER EIGHT

Allen, S., Basilio, I., Eraser, S., Stock, H., Garrison, W., Cohen, L., et al. (1994). Proximate traumatic sequelae of Hurricane Andrew on the police family. In J. Reese & E. Scrivner (Eds.), *Law enforcement families: Issues and answers*

(#1994-387-165/24333, pp. 143–154). Washington, DC: U.S. Department of Justice, Federal Bureau of Investigation, U.S. Government Printing Office.

Allison, D. (1992). *Bastard out of Carolina.* New York: Plume.

Chira, S. (1994, May 26). The benefits in emotional control. *New York Times.*

Everstine, D., & Everstine, L. (1993). *The trauma response: Treatment for emotional injury.* New York: Norton.

Johnson, K. (1989). *Trauma in the lives of children: Crisis and stress management techniques for teachers, counselors, and student service professionals.* Alameda, CA: Hunter House.

San Fernando Valley Child Guidance Clinic. (1986, July). *Coping with children's reactions to earthquakes and other disasters.* (Available from the author at 9650 Zelzah Avenue, Northridge, CA 91325)

Shuster, M., Stein, B., et al. (2001, November 15). A national survey of stress reactions after the September 11, 2001 terrorist attacks. *New England Journal of Medicine, 345*(20).

Sommers, G. (1991, May 20). On the front lines: Police stress and family well-being (45-659-0-91-1, pp. 7–10). Hearing before the Select Committee on Children, Youth, and Families, House of Representatives, 102nd Congress. Washington, DC: U.S. Government Printing Office.

Wee, D. (1994). Disasters: Impact on the law enforcement family. In J. Reese & E. Scrivner (Eds.), *Law enforcement families: Issues and answers* (#1994-387-165/24333, pp. 239-250). Washington, DC: U.S. Department of Justice, Federal Bureau of Investigation, U.S. Government Printing Office.

CHAPTER NINE

Attorney General's Task Force of Pennsylvania. (1989). *Domestic violence: A model protocol for police response.* Harrisburg, PA: Office of the Attorney General.

Bergen, G., Bourne-Lindamood, C., & Brecknock, S. (2000). Incidence of domestic violence among rural and small town law enforcement officers. In D. Sheehan (Ed.), *Domestic violence by police officers* (pp. 63–71). Washington, DC: U.S. Department of Justice, Federal Bureau of Investigation, U.S. Government Printing Office.

Boyd, L., Carlson, D., Smith. R., & Sykes, G. (1995). *Domestic assault among police: A survey of internal affairs policies.* Report prepared by Arlington, Texas, Police Department, and Southwestern Law Enforcement Institute. (Available from 817-459-5717)

Browne, A. (1987). *When battered women kill.* New York: Macmillan/Free Press.

Browne, A. (1993, October). Violence against women by male partners: Prevalence, outcomes and policy implications. *American Psychologist, 48*(10), 1077–1087.

Campion, M. (2000). Small police departments and police officer-involved domestic violence: A survey. In D. Sheehan (Ed.), *Domestic violence by police offi-*

cers (pp. 123–131). Washington, DC: U.S. Department of Justice, Federal Bureau of Investigation, U.S. Government Printing Office.

Chicago Police Department. (1996, February). Domestic violence: Our professional and personal response. *CPD Notebook, 2*(1), 2.

Countering violence at home. (1991, July 23). *Washington Post.*

D'Agostino, C., & Swann, G. (1994). Post shooting trauma and domestic violence: Clinical observation and preliminary data. In J. Reese & E. Scrivner (Eds.), *Law enforcement families: Issues and answers* (#1994-387-165/24333, pp. 227–232). Washington, DC: U.S. Department of Justice, Federal Bureau of Investigation, U.S. Government Printing Office.

Erwin, M., Gershon, R., Tiburzi, M., & Lin, S. (2005, February). Reports of intimate partner violence made against police officers. *Journal of Family Violence, 20*(1).

Feltgen, J. (1996, October). Domestic violence: When the abuser is a police officer. *Police Chief, LXIII,* 42–49.

Gallo, G. (2005, February). A family affair: Domestic violence in police families. *Police,* pp. 36–40.

Gershon, R. (1999, 2000). Police stress and domestic violence in police families in Baltimore, Maryland (1997/1999, computer file), ICPSR version. Baltimore: Johns Hopkins University [producer]. Ann Arbor, MI: Inter-university Consortium for Political and Social Research [distributor].

Gershon, R. (2000). National Institute of Justice final report, Project Shields (97-FS-VX-0001; available at www.ncjrs.gov).

Hanks, S. E. (1992). Treatment of maritally violent individuals. In E. C. Viano (Ed.), *Intimate violence: Interdisciplinary perspectives* (pp. 157–172). Washington, DC: Hemisphere.

Harway, M., & Hansen, M. (1994). *Spouse abuse: Assessing and treating battered women, batterers, and their children.* Sarasota, FL: Professional Resource Press.

Hays, G. (1994). Police couples: Breaking the security access code. In J. Reese & E. Scrivner (Eds.), *Law enforcement families: Issues and answers* (#1994-387-165/24333, pp. 337–344). Washington, DC: U.S. Department of Justice, Federal Bureau of Investigation, U.S. Government Printing Office.

Honig, A., & White, E. (1994). Violence and the law enforcement family. In J. Reese & E. Scrivner (Eds.), *Law enforcement families: Issues and answers* (#1994-387-165/24333, pp. 101–107). Washington, DC: U.S. Department of Justice, Federal Bureau of Investigation, U.S. Government Printing Office.

International Association of Police Chiefs. (2003, July). *Domestic violence by police officers: A policy of the IACP Police Response to Violence Against Women Project.* Available from the IACP, 515 North Washington Street, Alexandria, VA 22314; 800-THE-IACP, ext. 216.

Inwald, R., Traynor, W., & Favuzza, V. (2000). Psychological profiles of police and public safety officers accused of domestic violence. In D. Sheehan (Ed.), *Domestic violence by police officers* (pp. 209–224). Washington, DC: U.S. Department of Justice, Federal Bureau of Investigation, U.S. Government Printing Office.

Johnson, L. (1991, May 20). *On the front lines: Police stress and family well-being* (45-659-0-91-1). Hearing before the Select Committee on Children, Youth, and Families, House of Representatives, 102nd Congress. Washington, DC: U.S. Government Printing Office.

Johnson, M. (1995, May). Patriarchal terrorism and common couple violence: Two forms of violence against women. *Journal of Marriage and the Family, 57*(2), 283.

Johnson, M., & Roberts, M. Psychological History Questionnaire data 2001–2003. Personal communication.

Kruger, K. J., & Valltos, N. G. (2002, July). Dealing with domestic violence in law enforcement relationships. *FBI Law Enforcement Bulletin,* pp. 1–7.

Lott, L. (1995, November). Deadly secrets: Violence in the police family. *FBI Law Enforcement Bulletin,* pp. 12–16.

McKenry, P., Julian, T., & Gavazzi, S. (1995, May). Toward a biopsychosocial model of domestic violence. *Journal of Marriage and the Family, 57*(2), 307.

Marsella, A., Friedman, M., Gerrity, E., & Scurfield, R. (1996). *Ethnocultural aspects of posttraumatic stress disorder.* Washington, DC: American Psychological Association.

Martinez, J. (1994). *Hostages in the home: Domestic violence seen through its parallel, the Stockholm syndrome.* Unpublished manuscript.

National Center for Injury Prevention and Control: Center for Disease Control. Intimate partner violence: Fact sheet. www.cdc.gov/ncipc/factsheets/ipvfacts.html

National Center for Women and Policing. (2005). Police family violence fact sheet. www.womenandpolicing.org/violenceFS.asp

National Coalition against Domestic Violence. (1993). Facts on domestic violence. (Cited in *Crime and victimization in America: Statistic overview.* Washington, DC: National Victim Center.)

Neidig, P. H., & Freidman, D. H. (1984). *Spouse abuse: A treatment program for couples* (pp. 205–207). Champaign, IL: Research Press.

Neidig, P., Russell, H., & Seng, A. (1992, Spring). Interspousal aggression in law enforcement families: A preliminary investigation. *Police Studies, 15*(1), 30–38.

Neidig, P., Russell, H., & Seng, A. (1994). Observations and recommendations concerning the prevention and treatment of interspousal aggression in law enforcement families. In J. Reese & E. Scrivner (Eds.), *Law enforcement families: Issues and answers* (#1994-387-1657 24333, pp. 353–358). Washington, DC: U.S. Department of Justice, Federal Bureau of Investigation, U.S. Government Printing Office.

Pence, E., & Paymar, M. (1993). *Education groups for men who batter: The Duluth model.* New York: Springer.

Ryan, A. (2000). The prevalence of domestic violence in police families. In D. Sheehan (Ed.), *Domestic violence by police officers* (pp. 297–307). Washington, DC: U.S. Department of Justice, Federal Bureau of Investigation, U.S. Government Printing Office.

Schroeder, P. (1991, May 20). *On the front lines: Police stress and family well-being*

(45-659-0-91-1, p. 99). Hearing before the Select Committee on Children, Youth, and Families, House of Representatives, 102nd Congress. Washington, DC: U.S. Government Printing Office.

Sheehan, D. (2000). *Domestic violence in police officers*. Washington, DC: U.S. Department of Justice, Federal Bureau of Investigation, U.S. Government Printing Office.

Sonkin, D. J., & Durphy, M. (1989). *Learning to live without violence*. Volcano, CA: Volcano Press.

Stark, E. (1995). Representing woman battering: From battered woman syndrome to coercive control. *Albany Law Review, 58,* 973–1026.

Stith, S. (1990a). Police response to domestic violence: The influence of individual and familial factors. *Violence and Victims, 5*(1), 37–49.

Stith, S. (1990b). The relationship between the male police officer's response to victims of domestic violence and his personal and family experience. In E. C. Viano (Ed.), *The victimology handbook: Research findings, treatment, and public policy* (pp. 77–93). New York: Garland Press.

Stone, A. (2000). Domestic violence committed by law enforcement personnel: A fitness-for-duty approach. In D. Sheehan (Ed.), *Domestic violence by police officers* (pp. 323–330). Washington, DC: U.S. Department of Justice, Federal Bureau of Investigation, U.S. Government Printing Office.

Tolman, R. M., & Edelson, J. (1995). Interventions for men who batter: A review of research. In S. M. Stith & M. A. Straus (Eds.), *Understanding partner violence: Prevalence, causes, consequences, and solutions*. Minneapolis, MN: National Council on Family Relations.

U.S. Department of Justice: Bureau of Justice Statistics. Intimate partner violence 1993–2001. www.ojp.usdoj.gov/bjs/abstract/ipv01.htm and www.ojp.usdoj.gov/bjs/ub/ascii/fvs.txt.

Violence on the home front. (1995, September 13). *New York Post.*

Waits, K. (1985). The criminal justice system's response to battering: Understanding the problem, forging the solutions. *Washington Law Review, 267.* (Cited in S. Buel, S. Groisser, & M. Marryman. [1991, September]. *Harvard Law School battered women's advocacy project training and resource manual.*)

Walton, S., & Zelig, M. (2000). Whatever he does, don't fight back or you'll lose your gun: Strategies police officer victims use to cope with spousal abuse. In D. Sheehan (Ed.), *Domestic violence by police officers* (pp. 365–373). Washington, DC: U.S. Department of Justice, Federal Bureau of Investigation, U.S. Government Printing Office.

CHAPTER TEN

Al-Anon. (1980). *Are you troubled by someone's drinking?* (Available from Al-Anon Family Group Headquarters, Virginia Beach, VA)

Al-Anon. (1994). *What do YOU do about the alcoholic's drinking?* (P-19). (Available from Al-Anon Family Group Headquarters, Virginia Beach, VA)

Al-Anon. (1995). So *you love an alcoholic* (P-14). (Available from Al-Anon Family Group Headquarters, Virginia Beach, VA)

Allen, S. (1986). Suicide and indirect self-destructive behavior among police. In J. Reese & H. Goldstein (Eds.), *Psychological services for law enforcement* (85-600538, pp. 413–417). Washington, DC: U.S. Government Printing Office.

Allen, S. (1995, August). *The dynamics of suicide.* Unpublished paper, APA Police Psychology Mini Convention, New York.

Aussant, G. (1984). Police suicide. *R.C.M.P. Gazette, 46*(5), 14–21.

Aadmodt, M. G., & Stalnaker, N. A. (2001). Police officer suicide: Frequency and officer profiles. In D. C. Shehan & J. I. Warren (Eds.), *Suicide and law enforcement* (pp. 383–398). Washington, DC: Federal Bureau of Investigation.

Black, C. (1979). *My dad loves me, my dad has a disease.* Denver, CO: MAC.

Black, C. (1982). *It will never happen to me.* Denver, CO: MAC.

Blau, T. H. (1994). *Psychological services for law enforcement.* New York: Wiley.

Corelli, R. (1994, March 28). Booze and the badge. *Maclean's, 107,* 52.

D'Angelo, J. (1994). Alcoholism and chemical dependency in law enforcement: Its effects on the officer and the family members. In J. Reese & E. Scrivner (Eds.), *Law enforcement families: Issues and answers* (#1994-387-165/24333, pp. 57–66). Washington, DC: U.S. Department of Justice, Federal Bureau of Investigation, U.S. Government Printing Office.

Danieli, Y. (1994). Trauma to the family: Intergenerational sources of vulnerability and resilience. In J. Reese & E. Scrivner (Eds.), *Law enforcement families: Issues and answers* (#1994-387-165/24333, pp. 163–171). Washington, DC: U.S. Department of Justice, Federal Bureau of Investigation, U.S. Government Printing Office.

Gelles, M. (1995). Psychological autopsy: An investigative aid. In M. I. Kurke & E. M. Scrivner (Eds.), *Police psychology into the 21st century* (pp. 337-356). Hillsdale, NJ: Erlbaum.

Gilbert, R. (1986). A coordinated approach to alcoholism treatment. In J. T. Reese & H. A. Goldstein (Eds.), *Psychological services for law enforcement* (85-600538, pp. 115–120). Washington, DC: U.S. Government Printing Office.

Glossick, J. (1988, October). Don't let a good cop go bad: Chemical dependency is treatable. *Police Chief, LV*(10), 38.

Gross-Farina, S. (1993, March). Fit for duty?: Cops, choir practice and another chance for healing. *University of Miami Law Review, 47*(4), 1110–1111.

Horvitz, L. (1994, November 7). Can police solve their epidemic of suicide? *Insight on the News, 10*(45), 9.

Ivanoff, A. (1994, October 17). Police suicide. Testimony to the New York City Council.

Janik, J. (1995, January). Who needs peer support? *Police Chief, LXII*(1), 38–41.

Janik, J., & Kravitz, H. (1994). Police suicides: Trouble at home. In J. T. Reese & E. M. Scrivner (Eds.), *Law enforcement families: Issues and answers* (#1994-387-165/24333, pp. 73–81). Washington, DC: U.S. Department of Justice, Federal Bureau of Investigation, U.S. Government Printing Office.

Kaiser Permanente Medical Care Program. (1988). *Thinking about alcohol and drugs.* (Available from Kaiser Permanente, Oakland, CA)

Kaiser Permanente Healthwise Handbook. (1994). Boise, ID: Healthwise.

Kirschman, E. (1983). Wounded heroes: A case study and systems analysis of job-related stress and emotional dysfunction in three police officers. *Dissertation Abstracts International* (University Microfilms, no. 83-19, 921).

Lerner, H. (1989). *The dance of intimacy.* New York: Harper & Row.

Marzuk, P. M., Nock, M. K., Leon, A. C., Portera, L., & Tardiff, K. (2001, December). Suicide among New York City police officers, 1977–1996. *American Journal of Psychiatry, 159,* 2069–2071.

Maslach, C., & Jackson, S. (1979). Burned out cops and their families. *Psychology Today, 12*(12), 58–62.

McCafferty, F. (1992). Stress and suicide in police officers. *Southern Medical Journal, 85,* 233–243.

McKay, M., Davis, M., & Fanning, P. (1983). *Messages: The communications skills book.* Oakland, CA: New Harbinger.

Mills, J. W. (1982). *Coping with stress: A guide to living.* New York: Wiley.

North, C. S.. Tivis, L., McMillen, J. C., Pfefferbaum, B., Cox, J., Spitznagel, E. L., et al. (2002). Coping, functioning and adjustment of rescue workers after the Oklahoma City bombing. *Journal of Traumatic Stress, 15*(3), 171–175.

Pendergrass, V., & Ostrove, N. (1986). Correlates of alcohol use by police personnel. In J. T. Reese & H. A. Goldstein (Eds.), *Psychological services for law enforcement* (85-600538, pp. 480–495). Washington, DC: U.S. Government Printing Office.

Powers, W. (1988, October). Work performance counseling with the alcoholic officer. *Police Chief, LV*(10), 92.

Schaef, A. W., & Fassel, D. (1988). *The addictive organization.* New York: Harper & Row.

Scrivner, E. M. (1991, May 20). *On the front lines: Police stress and family well-being* (45-659-0-91-1, p. 99). Hearing before the Select Committee on Children, Youth, and Families, House of Representatives, 102nd Congress. Washington, DC: U.S. Government Printing Office.

Seligman, J. (1994, September). Cops who kill—themselves. *Newsweek,* p. 58.

Shneidman, E. S. (1985). *Definition of suicide.* New York: Wiley.

Skultety, S., & Singer, R. (1994). Choir practice and the family. In J. Reese & E. Scrivner (Eds.), *Law enforcement families: Issues and answers* (#1994-387-165/24333, pp. 83–89). Washington, DC: U.S. Department of Justice, Federal Bureau of Investigation, U.S. Government Printing Office.

Tighe, M., & Ivanoff, A. (1992). *Suicide and the police officer: Getting help before it's too late.* Instructor's manual for *By their own hand,* a film about police suicide. (Produced by the New York City Police Foundations, Inc., 345 Park Avenue, New York, NY 10154-0037; 1-212-751-8170; $75)

Violanti, J. M. (1996). *Police suicide: Epidemic in blue.* Springfield, IL: Thomas.

Violanti, J., Vena, J., Marshall, J., & Petrallia, S. (1996, Spring). Comparative evaluation of police suicide rate validity. *Journal of Suicide and Life-Threatening Behavior, 26*(1), 79–85.

Wagner, M., & Brzeczek, R. (1983, August). Alcoholism and suicide: A fatal connection. *FBI Law Enforcement Bulletin,* 8–15.

Waters, J. (2002). Moving ahead from September 11: A stress/crisis/trauma response model. *Brief Treatment and Crisis Intervention, 2*(1), 55–74.

Waters, J. *The trauma of September 11.* Unpublished article, available from the author at Fairleigh Dickinson University, Madison, NJ 07940, or judithawaters @aol.com.

CHAPTER ELEVEN

American Psychological Association. (1992, December). Ethical principles of psychologists and code of conduct. *American Psychologist, 47*(12), 1597–1611.

Archibald, E. (1995). Managing professional concerns in the delivery of psychological services to the police. In M. I. Kurke & E. M. Scrivner (Eds.), *Police psychology into the 21st century* (pp. 45–54). Hillsdale, NJ: Erlbaum.

Department of Consumer Affairs. (n.d.). *Professional therapy never includes sex.* (Available from the author at 1020 N Street, Sacramento, CA 95814)

Drug vs. talk therapy. (2004, October). Consumer Reports.org.

Everstine, D., & Everstine, L. (1993). *The trauma response: Treatment for emotional injury.* New York: Norton.

Gross-Farina, S. (1990). *Counseling: The ins and outs (A guide for law enforcement officers).* Out of print.

Gund, N., & Elliott, B. (1995). Employee assistance programs in police organizations. In M. I. Kurke & E. M. Scrivner (Eds.), *Police psychology into the 21st century* (pp. 149–168). Hillsdale, NJ: Erlbaum.

Horvitz, L. (1994, November 7). Can police solve their epidemic of suicide? *Insight on the News,* p. 9.

Kirschman, E. (1995). Organization consultation to law enforcement. In M. I. Kurke & E. M. Scrivner (Eds.), *Police psychology into the 21st century* (pp. 375–390). Hillsdale, NJ: Erlbaum.

Mental health: Does therapy help? (1995, November). *Consumer Reports,* pp. 734–739.

Walima, S., & Kirschman, E. (1988, October). Health resource coordinators: Organization consultation services. *Police Chief, LV*(10), 78–81.

CHAPTER TWELVE

Balkin, J. (1988). Why policemen don't like policewomen. *Journal of Police Science and Administration, 16*(1), 29–38.

Bouza, A. V. (1990). *The police mystique: An insider's look at cops, crime and the criminal justice system.* New York: Plenum Press.

Brown, J. M., & Campbell, E. A. (1994). *Stress and policing.* London: Wiley.

Brown, M. C. (1994, September). The plight of female police: A survey of NW patrolmen. *Police Chief, LX*(9), 50–53.

Buhrke, R. A. (1996). *A matter of justice: Lesbians and gay men in law enforcement*. New York: Routledge.

Cooper, C. (1992, January 5). Women cops taking on harassment fight. *San Francisco Examiner*.

Curran, S. (1994). Sexual harassment of the female officer: Effects on the police family. In J. T. Reese & E. M. Scrivner (Eds.), *Law enforcement families: Issues and answers* (#1994-387-165/24333, pp. 271–274). Washington, DC: U.S. Department of Justice, Federal Bureau of Investigation, U.S. Government Printing Office.

Daum, J., & Johns, C. M. (1994, September). Police work from a woman's perspective. *Police Chief, LXI*(9), 46–49.

Debro, J. (1993, March). Stress and its control: A minority perspective. *Police Chief, LX*(3).

Fletcher, C. (1995). *Breaking and entering: Women cops talk about life in the ultimate men's club*. New York: HarperCollins.

Greene, R. L. (1987). Psychological support for women entering law enforcement. In H. W. More & P. Unsinger (Eds.), *Police managerial use of psychology and psychologists* (pp. 171–187). Springfield, IL: Thomas.

Hochschild, A. B. (1986). *The second shift*. New York: Viking.

Johnson, L. B. (1989, Winter). The employed black: The dynamics of work–family tension. *Review of Black Political Economy, 17*(3), 69–85.

Johnson, L. B. (1991). Job strain among police officers: Gender comparison. *Police Studies, 14*(12–16), 107–113.

Johnson, L. B. (1995). Gender comparisons. In W. G. Bailey (Ed.), *The encyclopedia of police science* (2nd ed., pp. 591–598). New York: Garland.

Johnson, L. B., Nieva, V., & Wilson, M. J. (1985, Winter). *Police work/home stress study: Interim report*. Rockville, MD: National Institute of Mental Health.

Jones, J. W.(1995). Counseling issues and police diversity. In M. Kurke & E. M. Scrivner (Eds.), *Police psychology into the 21st century* (pp. 207–254). Hillsdale, NJ: Erlbaum.

Kanter, R. M. (1977). *Men and women of the corporation*. New York: Basic Books.

Kanter, R. M. [Producer]. (1980). *A tale of "O": On being different* [Video]. (Available from Goodmeasure, Inc., Boston, MA 02142)

Katz, J. (1994, July 11). The myth of rampant police brutality. *New York Magazine*, pp. 39–40.

Kay, S. (1994, September). Why women don't apply to be police officers. *Police Chief, LX*(9), 44–45.

Leinen, S. (1993). *Gay cops*. New Brunswick, NJ: Rutgers University Press.

Martin, S. E. (1980). *Breaking and entering: Police women on patrol*. Berkeley: University of California Press.

McDowell, J. (1992, February 17). Are women better cops? *Time*, pp. 70–72.

McNaught, B. (1993). *Gay issues in the workplace*. New York: St. Martin's Press.

Ness, C., & Gordon, R. (1995, August 19). Sisters on patrol. *San Francisco Examiner*, p. A-ll.

Niederhoffer, A., & Niederhoffer, E. (1978). *The police family: From station house to ranch house.* Lexington, MA: Lexington Books.

Poole, E., & Pogrebin, M. (1988). Factors affecting the decision to remain in policing: A study of women officers. *Journal of Police Science and Administration, 16*(1), 49–55.

Quinn, V. (1981). *Policewomen and role conflict: A literature survey.* Unpublished paper.

Skolnick, J. H. (1966). *Justice without trial: Law enforcement in a democratic society.* New York: Wiley.

Stewart, C. (1995). *Comprehensive program and instructional model for training on socially stigmatized communities.* (Available from the author at 710 West 27th Street, #10, Los Angeles, CA 90007; 213-749-1443)

Wexler, J. G., & Quinn, V. (1985, June). Considerations in the training and development of women sergeants. *Journal of Police Science and Administration, 13*(2), 98–105.

CHAPTERS THIRTEEN AND FOURTEEN

Beehr, T., Johnson, L., & Nieva, R. (1995). Occupational stress of police and their spouses. *Journal of Organizational Behavior, 1*(16), 3–25.

Bernard, J. (1972). *The future of marriage.* New York: World Publishers.

Boorstein, S., (1995). *It's easier than you think.* New York: HarperCollins.

Borum, R., & Philpot, C. (1993). Therapy with law enforcement couples: Clinical management of the high risk lifestyle. *American Journal of Family Therapy, 21*(2)., 122–135.

Bradstreet, R. (1994). Cultural hurdles to healthy police families. In J. Reese & E. Scrivner (Eds.), *Law enforcement families: Issues and answers* (#1994-387-165/24333, pp. 19–26). Washington, DC: U.S. Department of Justice, Federal Bureau of Investigation, U.S. Government Printing Office.

Chance, S. (1988, June). Partners in life. *Police,* pp. 32–35.

Gilmartin, K. (1990). The brotherhood of biochemistry: Its implications for a police career. In H. E. Russell & A. Beigel (Eds.), *Understanding human behavior for effective police work* (3rd ed., pp. 397–418). New York: Basic Books.

Lerner, H. G. (1989). *The dance of intimacy: A woman's guide to courageous acts of change in key relationships.* New York: Harper & Row.

Proulx, E. A. (1993). *The shipping news.* New York: Simon & Schuster.

Schmuckler, E. (1994). The dual career family in law enforcement: A concern for management. In J. T. Reese & E. M. Scrivner (Eds.), *Law enforcement families: Issues and answers* (#1994-387-165/24333, pp. 41–50). Washington, DC: U.S. Department of Justice, Federal Bureau of Investigation, U.S. Government Printing Office.

Wallerstein, J. S., & Blakeslee, S. (1995). *The good marriage: How and why love lasts.* Boston: Houghton Mifflin.

INDEX

Index

Avoidance
    family support and, 138
    posttraumatic stress disorder (PTSD) and, 104, 105
    as a reaction to critical incident stress, 94, 95
    responses of children to trauma and, 154

Battered Women's Support Services, 298
Bedtime troubles in children, 152–153
Behavioral signs of critical incident stress
    overview, 94
    responses of children to trauma and, 151, 155
Beliefs, core, 122–123
Beside the Badge, 289
Betty Ford Center, 295
Biochemistry of trauma, 97–100
Biofeedback, 120
Bioterrorism, 93
Blood pressure, 94
Bottles and Badges, 194
Bottom line, alcohol use and, 192, 194–195
Breathing difficulties, 94
British Association for Counseling and Psychotherapy, 283, 293
British Association for Women Police (BAWP), 300–301
Bureaucratic nature of police work
    overview, 65–66
    second injury and, 74–78
    See also Organizational stress

Canadian Centre for Emergency Preparedness, 294
Canadian Police Wives, 293
Canadian Psychological Association (CPA), 283
Canadian Traumatic Stress Network, 285
Care of Police Survivors (COPS), 288
Career management
    applicant phase, 43–45
    crossroad phase, 58–62
    disillusionment phase, 54–58
    honeymoon phase, 47–51
    rookie officers, 45–47
    settling down phase, 51–53
    tips for, 62–63
Catastrophizing
    controlling nature of police work and, 36
    minority officers and, 239
Centre for Suicide Prevention, 288–289
Chest pains, 94
Chiefs of police, stress and, 55
Child abuse, confidentiality and, 210
Childhood experiences of officers
    critical incident stress and, 101–102
    risk factors for PTSD and, 103
Children, death of, 93
Children of a police officer
    controlling nature of police work and, 36
    cop couples and, 242, 252–253, 255–257
    delayed reactions of, 148–149
    domestic violence and, 174

    emotional expression and, 145–147
    family support and, 137
    information regarding incidents and, 148
    overview, 142–143
    professional help and, 214
    providing a safe haven for, 143–150
    public scrutiny and, 21–22
    reassurance of, 144–145
    resources for, 289–294
    responses to trauma, 150–155
    tips for helping deal with crisis, 156
    trauma and, 134–136
    when to pursue professional help for, 155
    See also Families of officers
Choir practice, 97, 112
Closure, recovery from trauma and, 127
Coaching children, 146–147
Cognitive-behavioral therapy (CBT), 119–120
Cognitive signs of critical incident stress, 95
Command presence, 34–38
Communication
    controlling nature of police work and, 36–38
    cop couples and, 249
    disciplinary action and, 74
    emotional control and, 31
    female officers and, 229
    during the honeymoon phase, 51
    long hours and, 18
    marital problems and, 215
    organizational stress and, 66
    protective factors against PTSD and, 108
    traumatic stress in the family and, 141
Community policing, 61–62
Compassion fatigue, 32
Compassion for others, 110
Compassionate Friends, 286
Compensation
    minority officers and, 241
    organizational stress and, 66
Competency, sense of
    female officers and, 229–230
    recovery from trauma and, 114
Competitiveness, 257
Concentration difficulties
    posttraumatic stress disorder (PTSD) and, 105
    as a reaction to critical incident stress, 95
Concerns of Police Survivors, Inc. (COPS), 286
Conduct disorders in children, 174
Confidentiality in treatment, 208–213
Confrontation, 36–38
Confusion, 95
Consultation, confidentiality and, 213
Control-related abuse, 172
Controlling nature of police work
    cop couples and, 257
    domestic violence and, 166, 172, 180
    overview, 34–38
    personality commonalities and, 44
COP-2-COP, 280–281
Cop couples
    examples of, 243–254
    overview, 242
    tips for, 255–257

Index

Index

Index

335

Index

Index

Index

ABOUT THE AUTHOR

Ellen Kirschman, PhD, is a clinical psychologist and consultant who works with peace officers and their families. She has written extensively about police culture and is sought after as a speaker and seminar leader. Dr. Kirschman has been an invited guest at the FBI Academy and is a member of the Psychological Services Sub-section of the International Association of Chiefs of Police. She is a cofounder of www.policefamilies.com and maintains a website for the public at www.ellenkirschman.com. In 2000, Dr. Kirschman was named Woman of Distinction by the Police Chiefs Spouses Worldwide. She lives in Redwood City, California.